GW01033847

RESILIENCE

Lessons from Sir William Wilde on Life after Covid

RESILIENCE

Lessons from Sir William Wilde on Life after Covid

BRENDAN KELLY

EASTWOOD BOOKS

First published 2023 by Books Ireland
Dublin, Ireland

www.eastwoodbooks.com

First edition

Eastwood Books
The Wordwell Group
Unit 9, 78 Furze Road
Sandyford
Dublin, Ireland

ISBN: 978-1-913934-56-9 (paperback)
ISBN: 978-1-916742-53-6 (ebook)

British Library Cataloguing in Publication Data.
A catalogue record for this book is available from the National Library of Ireland
and the British Library.

Typesetting and design by the Wordwell Group
Printed in Ireland by Sprint Print

CONTENTS

A note on language
Throughout this book, original language and terminology from the past and from various archives, reports and publications have been maintained, except where explicitly indicated otherwise. This reflects an attempt to optimise fidelity to historical sources and does not reflect an endorsement of the broader use of such terminology in contemporary settings.

Content advisory
This book discusses mental illness, self-harm, suicide and related matters in direct terms, in order to demystify, delineate and understand them better. For this reason, some readers might find certain sections distressing.

This book is dedicated to Regina, Eoin and Isabel

INTRODUCTION

I wake at 2 a.m. with the worst headache of my life. An infinity of hammers pound my skull from within and without. The pain is excruciating when I stay still. It is worse when I move.

I was fine when I went to bed at 10 p.m., but four hours later I hold my head in my hands, shiver with a fever and rock back and forth in a hotel room. I phone the reception desk and a staff member gives me paracetamol. I survive the night, and the following morning I test positive for Covid-19.

The irony here is deep. It is April 2023 and, despite working in a hospital right through the pandemic, I never contracted Covid-19. Today, the day I finally test positive for the virus, is the first day of a week of leave that I took to finalise this book—a reflection on Ireland's journey out of the worst of Covid-19 and what the pandemic might mean.

Instead of working on this manuscript or anything else, I limp home, thoroughly humbled by the virus, bluntly reminded of my place in the world and in desperate need of more paracetamol.

Covid-19 stole lives, stole time and stole our peace of mind. There was nothing good about it. While some commentators argued that the pandemic made us slow down, notice the world around us and value each other more, Covid-19 killed millions, disrupted the lives of millions more, tore families asunder and consigned us to two years of emergency living in the shadow of uncertainty and fear. Any potential benefits were obliterated by the devastation that the virus brought to the world.

Ireland's response to Covid-19 was remarkably similar to responses elsewhere—a changing mix of public health measures that were generally agreed in principle but varied in degree over time. Most governments provided public health advice about avoiding infection, placed certain restrictions on movement, changed health systems in radical ways and—when vaccines became available—rolled out vast programmes of inoculation on a scale never seen before. Most critics of government responses either (reasonably) questioned the balance of measures employed or (inadvertently) demonstrated why they were not in decision-making positions themselves, or (sometimes) both.

The variations between countries were differences of degree: some countries had more lockdowns, some kept their schools closed longer and others were better at delivering vaccines. These variations are to be expected; they do not mean that specific governments were wrong in their responses but rather that the pandemic affected different countries in different ways, depending on their pre-existing states of health, public infrastructure and general approaches to problems on this scale.

When you also consider the initial scientific uncertainty about the virus and the political imperative to provide steady leadership, governmental responses to Covid-19 start to seem like miracles of consistency and good sense.

Comparing across countries is difficult, but most moderately reliable comparisons rate Ireland's response as either average or somewhat above. As a psychiatrist, the psychological response to the pandemic and its aftermath is what interests me the most. During Covid-19, were we kind to each other? Were we traumatised? Were we strong? Were we all of these things and more?

And now, in 2023, as the acute emergency subsides in many countries, how has the pandemic changed us as individuals, mentally, emotionally and psychologically? As a society, have we forgotten the trauma and simply moved on?

Looking back, it is clear that our sense of time was impaired for much of the outbreak, both when it was happening and in retrospect. While our memories of this period are by no means blank, most of us don't have two years' worth of memories for the two-year period of the worst of the pandemic in Ireland. This is partly because less happened on a day-to-day basis at its peak (especially during lockdowns), partly because much that happened was repetitive (not least the daily news bulletins) and partly because of the way that we process memories following trauma.[1]

After a distressing event, the brain processes the resultant large amount of emotionally charged information in bursts. In extreme situations, this contributes to the flashbacks, nightmares and re-experiencing seen in post-traumatic stress disorder (PTSD). In other words, the load is too great for the brain to process at the time, so some parts of the memories are processed immediately, some are repressed for processing later and other parts are reactivated by triggers (conscious and unconscious) over time.

While it is not accurate to say that Ireland has PTSD as a result of Covid-19 or anything as simple as that, it is clear that processing takes time, that there are memory blanks now which might be filled later and that memories are often reawakened, sometimes as emotions, sometimes unexpectedly and sometimes painfully. Even so, it is important that we remember, despite our understandable desire to move on from this experience.[2]

This book is a reflection on these issues. It is my effort to make sense of what happened. We need to move on, but with an awareness of what we have been through, how it felt and what our next move might be. I hope this helps.

This book is some things and is not other things.

Here is what this book is. It is my account of five seasons spent in Dublin, from spring 2021 to spring 2022, as Ireland emerged from the worst of Covid-19. I am a psychiatrist, a medical doctor who specialises in mental illness, and I worked in Dublin throughout the pandemic. I am interested in medical history, so this book is also a reflection on Sir William Wilde, a prominent Victorian doctor who, as well as being Oscar's father, contributed hugely to our understanding of pandemics in Irish history. Never was Wilde more relevant than he is today. Finally, this book contains a great deal about coffee, just because I like coffee very much.[i] Apologies in advance for this.

Here is what this book is not. It is not a scientific analysis of Ireland's public health response to Covid-19.[ii] I am happy to leave that task to others who are vastly more knowledgeable and skilled than I am in that area.[3] Neither is this book a systematic analysis of Ireland's political response to the pandemic, which has been admirably analysed by others and will doubtless be picked over for years to come.[4] Finally, this book is not an effort to draw simple 'lessons' from a complex event such as a pandemic. Life is both too long and too short for bumper stickers. The 'lessons' discussed in Chapter 5 may or may not have been learned—probably not.

In short, this is a book about stolen time but also about time savoured. It is about sitting with the memory of an extraordinary period in our lives rather than forcing an interpretation on it. Above all, and largely thanks to Sir William Wilde, this book is about the value of history in reminding us that there is always a bigger story, a longer history and a common humanity that is deeper than we know, wiser than we think and kinder than we can ever imagine.

***

i   Possibly too much.
ii I completed a master's degree in epidemiology in 2004, but the pandemic quickly taught me that my dimly remembered tutorials were about as useful as the salsa classes I attended around the same time. Mind you, I dabbled in on-line salsa during the pandemic, so I did salvage something from that period in my life.

Dublin hums. People, birds, bicycles, cars, trams, trains. Compression, closeness, hope.

Over a million people squeeze into this small area in search of connection, community, coffee. I do not understand cities but always seek to live in them.

I stand outside No. 1 Merrion Square, one-time home of Sir William Wilde, doctor, scholar, writer and father of playwright Oscar. Wilde was a celebrated figure in nineteenth-century Dublin, his achievements touched by controversy in later life. The plaque on his Merrion Square residence, now the American College Dublin, lists many roles:

> Sir William Robert Willis Wilde, 1815–1876, aural [ear] and ophthalmic [eye] surgeon, archaeologist, ethnologist, antiquarian, biographer, statistician, naturalist, topographer, historian, folklorist, lived in this house from 1855 to 1876.

His gravestone in Mount Jerome Cemetery at Harold's Cross adds pomp:

> Sir William Wilde, MD FRCSI, Surgeon Oculist [eye doctor] to Her Majesty Queen Victoria, Chevalier of the Royal Swedish Order of The North Star, the Founder of St Mark's Ophthalmic Hospital and the Author of Many Works Illustrative of the History and Antiquities of Ireland. Born at Castlerea, County Roscommon, March 1815. Died at his Residence, Merrion Square, Dublin, April 1876.

Wilde lived at 1 Merrion Square from 1855, the year after Oscar's birth, until his death at 4pm on 19 April 1876. He died, after a period of decline, in a second-floor room overlooking the historic square.[5] Today, a statue of Oscar slouches on a large stone in direct sight of the house, its vivid colours contrasting with the stolid elegance of the building in which Oscar grew up and where William saw patients and, eventually, died.

William and Oscar had a great deal in common. In 1976, on the centenary of William's death, Peter Froggatt of Queen's University, Belfast, spoke about William's 'exuberant, restless and eclectic mind, unrestrained and amorphous in so many ways'.[6] Froggatt's words might equally apply to Oscar, along with much of his description of William's work: 'Dynamic, exuberant, sound, ingenious, laborious, cautious, scientific and deserving of high accolade; but not quite flawless judged on the strictest criteria'.[7] Oscar's brilliance and flaws are no longer in dispute. Oscar's life, like William's, combined achievement with tribulation, although he was less 'cautious' than William (and virtually everyone else).

Today, in the era of Covid-19, I am drawn to Wilde's Dublin home not by William's storied life or Oscar's wit but by a specific aspect of William's work which obsessed him in the 1850s: 'I gave up all society and recreation for 18 months,' he wrote, 'and more than once … impaired my health by the incessant daily and nightly labour devoted to this voluminous work.'[8] This 'work' cemented William Wilde's reputation as a brilliant medical mind, earned him a knighthood in 1864 and fascinates me today as Ireland emerges from the Covid-19 pandemic, blinking in the light.

From November 1854 to May 1856 Wilde devoted himself to analysing the results of the Irish national census of 1851, the most detailed population census undertaken to that point. Building on his involvement in the 1841 census, he scrutinised, studied and tabulated the 1851 results with unparalleled clarity. He interpreted findings, drew conclusions and applied lessons. He wrote at length, put the census numbers into context, explored their historical background and brought his deep knowledge of Irish society to bear on what would in other hands have proved a dry statistical exercise. William Wilde was anything but dry.

The results of the 1851 census were published in ten volumes totalling 4,533 pages. Wilde single-handedly wrote two of those volumes, Parts III and V.[9] Part III was a 150-page 'Report on the Status of Disease', in which Wilde quantified the challenges presented by 'the deaf and dumb', 'the blind', 'the lunatic and idiotic', 'the lame and decrepit', and 'the sick' in workhouses, hospitals, prisons and asylums.[10] He had a broad understanding of the social impact of illness, which brought much-needed nuance to his analysis of the census.

Wilde presented Part V of the census in two volumes, collectively called 'Tables of Deaths'. The grim title conceals a multitude of wonders and has direct relevance to Covid-19.

The first volume of Part V amounts to 560 pages and includes a 270-page 'Table of Cosmical Phenomena, Epizootics, Famines, and Pestilences in Ireland'.[11] Wilde starts this epic account in the 'Pagan or Pre-Christian Period' and recounts a bewildering array of illnesses, misfortunes and bizarre celestial events up to 1851.[12] These were the Covid-19s of their eras.

The breadth of Wilde's reports is astonishing, their detail extraordinary, their vision inspiring and occasionally apocalyptic. To take random examples, this table records a 'great famine' during the reign of Cairbre, the 'Cat-headed' high king of Ireland in AD 10, as well as St Patrick treating a leper's sores 'with his own hands' in 432, and various extraordinary occurrences in 688, recorded in detail in the *Annals of Clonmacnoise*: 'It rained blood in Leinster this year; butter was turned into the colour of blood; and a wolf was seen and heard speak with human voice'.[13]

Blood and mass destruction feature repeatedly. In 806, 'cakes were converted into blood, and the blood flowed from them when being cut', according to the *Annals of the Four Masters*.[14] In 960, 'an arrow of fire came from the south-west along Leinster, and killed hundred thousands of men and cattle, with the houses of Dublin burned'.[15] There was plenty of bad weather, too, including 'snow beyond measure' in 766 and 'great rains' in August 1817, resulting in damaged crops and widespread illness: 'Fever spread through the north in September. Kilkenny was next attacked, and Wicklow towards the end of the month. The disease then extended to Derry and Armagh.'[16] There were infections everywhere: Covid before Covid.

Wilde's accounts of ancient epidemics are especially arresting and relevant today. He starts with Ireland's 'first recorded pestilence' in *Tamlacht Muintire Parthaloin* (Tallaght) in 'the year of the world 2820, according to the long chronology of the Septuagint' (approximately 2680 BC).[17] He tells of a plague of *Baccach* (lameness) and dysentery in 708, a 'great pestilence' in 824, 'a great leprosy' and 'running of blood' in Dublin in 950, another 'great pestilence (*Teidhm*) over all Europe' in 1095, and a seemingly endless succession of other plagues, epidemics and illnesses to beset Ireland over the centuries.[18]

I am drawn to William Wilde today because his insights into Ireland's medical past and previous epidemics feel more urgent than ever. Wilde studied these phenomena, knew what he was talking about, had a lot to say.

Moreover, history matters. In 1864 Wilde published a lecture that he delivered to the Young Men's Christian Association on the subject of *Ireland, Past and Present: The Land and the People*.[19] With scant regard for his audience, he opened his talk by bemoaning their presumed ignorance of history:

How few there are in this vast assemblage of educated persons who know anything about the early history and antiquities of their native land![20]

Wilde, by contrast, was steeped in history, folklore and medicine. This makes him an excellent, if eccentric, guide to the present moment, as the Covid-19 pandemic subsides in Ireland and we ponder its impact on our worlds, our lives, our stories.

That is what this book is about: five seasons in Dublin, starting in spring 2021 as Ireland begins its journey out of the pandemic, and five lessons from Sir William Wilde, starting with his reflections on ancient epidemics and pestilence in Ireland.

That is all to come. For now, I stand alone outside Sir William's home at 1 Merrion Square, reading the plaque that commemorates Wilde senior. I ignore the scattering of tourists at the statue of Oscar across the road. William is the person for this moment in history.

When the plaque to William was unveiled here in 1971, a small crowd of scholars and enthusiasts gathered to celebrate the great man.[21] They stood where I stand now, forming a small huddle, wrapped in trench coats and speaking Irish in the driving rain. Two gardaí approached the group, ready to take names at what seemed, by all appearances, to be a commemorative meeting of an illegal organisation, maybe even a paramilitary one. The gardaí were not easy to dissuade, but eventually they left.

There are no such issues today. I leave in peace and solitude, in search of coffee. Dublin has twice as many coffee-shops per head of population as Prague, and four times as many as Paris.[22] I find a double espresso that strips my throat and fills my veins with thunder.

I might have a problem with coffee.

1. SPRING 2021: PLAGUE

'True wisdom comes to each of us when we realise how little we understand about life, ourselves, and the world around us.'

—*Socrates*

*T*his chapter starts in January 2021, as Ireland's Covid-19 vaccination programme commences. It feels like spring has come early. From February to May, I reflect on the start of the pandemic and its arrival in Ireland in February 2020. Since then, the year of loss, anxiety, lockdowns and endless statistics felt unprecedented but, in truth, was not new. It was only new to us. In his 1856 census report, William Wilde outlined the many plagues, famines and misfortunes that beset Ireland over the centuries, including (in his words) 'great waves of pestilence which had already passed (according to the general course of plagues) from the East, over the European continent, frequently carried along the track of human intercourse, by commercial dealings, or borne onward by hostile navies or invading armies'. Covid-19 is the most recent event in this long list of calamities. Its arrival is a fierce reminder of one of our *darker human destinies: infection, illness, death. A pandemic is elemental. The threat is everywhere and invisible. And yet spring 2021 brings hope in the form of vaccines. The scientists have delivered; it is up to politicians and societies to distribute vaccines fairly. This is a welcome challenge, but a challenge nonetheless.*

JANUARY 2021

January is named after Janus, the two-faced Roman god. Janus could see the past and the future. He represents beginnings, so January is a time of renewal and fresh challenges. In The Winter's Tale, *Shakespeare's Perdita says: 'You'd be so lean that blasts of January would blow you through and through. Now, my fair'st friend, I would I had some flowers o' the spring that might become your time of day; and yours, and yours.' In January 2021, Perdita's longed-for 'flowers o' the spring' have not yet arrived. We still endure the 'blasts' of winter winds, but change, perhaps, is in the air.*

At first, I do not recognise the feeling. It is distantly familiar, but its name escapes me.

It is 11 a.m. on Tuesday 5 January 2021. I stand at the door of the staff vaccination centre in Tallaght University Hospital, waiting for my Covid-19 vaccination.[1] I work in Tallaght as a psychiatrist, a medical doctor who specialises in mental illness.

A nurse beckons me in and explains the process. I sign a consent form. The nurse smiles.

I go to the next desk, where another nurse tells me how she will administer the vaccine. She answers my questions. She smiles.

Suddenly, I recognise the feeling in the room, the emotion I felt on arriving but struggled to name. It is hope.

No wonder I am confused.[i]

For almost a year now, I have seen my colleagues in the hospital work at the coalface of this pandemic. I witnessed the dedication of staff in our intensive care unit and medical wards as they treated the sickest patients with Covid-19 and other illnesses. I saw the fearlessness of our emergency department staff as they navigated the ever-changing face of the pandemic.

I admired the work of hospital management as they adapted hospital systems to an unprecedented challenge and created a vast vaccination programme. Their work is momentous. And I saw, firsthand, my colleagues in psychiatry provide mental health care to the most vulnerable. Never was it needed more.

Most of all, I witnessed the compassion of doctors, nurses, allied health professionals, cleaners, caterers and so many others who came to work every day, put on their personal protective equipment (PPE) and simply got the job done. These inspiring people never lost hope, even in the darkest days of this pandemic. In general practice and public health, too, the work has been exceptional.

i   I am confused quite often, if I am honest, but this was different.

As a country, our hope took a battering over the past year, since Ireland's first identified case of Covid-19 in February 2020. Case numbers rose inexorably. Restrictions tightened. Public frustration was palpable: when would all of this end? It was easy to lose hope.

But all of this *will* end. Pandemics pass. The losses are substantial but, as a country, we will come through this.

Our behaviour is our strongest defence. We have more power than we think.

We stay at home as much as possible. When we go out, we physically distance and wear face-coverings when appropriate. We stay apart and find new ways to connect.

Of course, certain restrictions are still in place as I write these words, on my vaccination day in January 2021, but the situation feels radically different because we have the prospect of a vaccine to sustain us. Roll-out will be careful but steady. The vaccines have passed all the safety checks. They are powerful tools. And safe.

What was that first vaccination like for me?

After so many months of build-up, the jab itself is an anticlimax. I barely feel it. It is less of a jab than the annual 'flu jab. 'Is that it?', I ask the nurse, somewhat deflated by the lack of drama. 'That's it', she says. 'You're done.'

I am observed for fifteen minutes to see whether I have an anaphylactic reaction. I do not. Five minutes later, I'm back at work. Over the following days, I watch for side-effects. I have none. The second dose, some weeks later, is similar: a quick jab and no side-effects whatsoever. It is as if nothing happened.

But something amazing did happen. I was vaccinated against Covid-19, the cause of the pandemic. It is always a privilege to work in healthcare, but now I was doubly privileged to be vaccinated too, at the very start of the vaccination programme.

Vaccines are what make January 2021 radically different to February 2020. They add that extra dollop of hope that makes all the difference.

After my vaccination, the hospital photographer takes a picture of me and the nurse who vaccinated me. 'For social media', he says.

In the photo, our faces are partially covered with masks, but it is clear that, despite the suffering of this pandemic, despite the losses and despite the hard weeks behind us and the tough months ahead, we are smiling.

They are tentative smiles, but they are smiles nonetheless, filled with hope. It is spring.

FEBRUARY 2021

'February' comes from the Latin word februum, *meaning purification.* Februa, *the Roman purification ritual, was held on the 15th of the month. February is a time of stormy transition, as spring approaches but winter is reluctant to leave. In Shakespeare's* Much Ado About Nothing, *Don Pedro asks Benedick: 'Why, what's the matter that you have such a February face, so full of frost, of storm and cloudiness?' Eventually, the frost, storm and cloudiness clear,*

we are purified of winter and spring officially arrives, in March.

Since childhood, I believed that February was the first month of spring. This year, I felt that my spring started in January, with vaccination. But, in my heart of hearts, I thought that spring truly arrived in February.

I liked this idea because, if spring commenced in February, it meant that autumn began in August. My birthday is in August. I have always felt like an autumn person, fond of the shorter evenings and the growing dark. I tolerate summer, love autumn and am happy enough in winter. Spring can go either way.

None of this matters, though, because I was wrong. Spring does not begin in February, let alone January. Spring begins in March. This news came as a blow when I first heard it. Who knew? Not I.[ii]

It turns out that I was wrong about many things, including (but not limited to) my childhood assumptions that spring began in February, that everyone loved chips, that everyone watched *Chips* on TV, and that life would continue forever as it was, undisrupted by natural disasters such as global pandemics.[iii]

---

ii Literally everyone else knew. While the traditional Irish calendar saw spring commence in February and autumn in August, general consensus is that spring starts in March and autumn in September. Everyone else knows this, it seems.

iii It turns out that the TV programme's real name was *CHiPs*, with a small 'i' and small 's' (weirdly). *CHiPs* was a crime series that ran

I was mistaken on all four counts. Not only does spring start in March but also, on a random Thursday afternoon when I was nine, Niall O'Toole shocked all of Third Class by announcing that he did not like chips—he preferred *rice*, of all things. At home, I stopped watching *CHiPs* when I was around 12, although I still look to it for life lessons, happiness hacks and kick-ass biking boots. Maybe some things do last forever.[iv]

Most of all, though, and on an entirely different scale, Covid-19 arrived in our lives in 2020 and shattered any residual child-like fantasies of permanence and inviolability. Suddenly, nothing felt safe anymore. It was as if everything could somehow suddenly end. And, for more than 2.6 million people in that terrible first year, it did.[2]

Covid-19 changed world-views forever, especially in rich countries. Up to then, this generation's experience was that serious disruptions belonged in places that were distant from Ireland and other wealthy western nations. Floods, volcanoes, earthquakes and plagues simply did not happen *here*. How could we see this coming? Might it have been predicted?

When I became a doctor in 1996, I was dimly aware that scientists continuously forecasted the arrival of new

from 1977 to 1983 in the US. It presumably arrived in Ireland some years later. The show featured two motorcycle officers in the California Highway Patrol (I see *now*: *CHiPs*). Growing up in the deep west of Ireland, I identified immediately with the two tough Americans.

iv   If you're wondering how *Chips* became *CHiPs*, see previous footnote.

infections that could spread across Europe and wreak havoc on our health, our lives and our societies. But scientists were *always* predicting that this would happen. Each year, virologists presented reasons why this year's predictions were more accurate than previous ones—and each year they were wrong.

People have always prophesied doom. If the core of the earth opens today and a herd of fire-breathing dragons appear, we will find someone who predicted that this precise event would occur in this specific way on this exact day. Hopefully, that person also has a plan for dealing with it.[v]

There was no systematic way of knowing that, in late December 2019, a new coronavirus, Covid-19, would be identified in China and would quickly spread around the world.[3] Inevitably, randomly, the predictions of a small number of people turned out to be correct. If their voices had been heeded at the time, things *might* have turned out differently (although more probably not). But while a stopped clock is right twice a day, mostly it is wrong. It was impossible to distinguish the few correct predictions from the many incorrect ones. The signal was lost in an infinity of noise. Perhaps it always is.

In early February 2020, as the scale of the outbreak became apparent, *The Guardian* commented that dealing 'with uncertainty and nuance is hard' but 'necessary if we are to act humanely and sensibly'.[4] Statistics emerging from

v   I doubt it.

China and elsewhere were not reassuring and did not assist with the search for certainty:

> Despite tens of millions being under lockdown in Hubei, around 640 people are dead and more than 31,500 infected (the vast majority in the Chinese province, but with other cases from Canada to Singapore to Russia). It is unpredictable: we remain unsure of its transmissibility and its fatality rate. We do not know how far it has spread already. We do not know whether it will be containable … What is needed is the best response, not the toughest: scalpels rather than hammers.

Today, over a year later, sitting by the Grand Canal in Dublin at 6 a.m. in late February 2021, I am sleepless and exhausted after a year of rolling news about the pandemic. If anything, I have heard too many statistics. I no longer know what to make of them (if I ever did).

Both 'scalpels' and 'hammers' have been used to contain this virus, but it is almost impossible to know how effective these measures have been. The situation could be worse, for sure, but could it be better? Is there any way to tell?

Right now, in the early morning, everything seems peaceful. Dublin sleeps. Is anyone else up? Wakeful mid-pandemic, checking their phones for news? Or maybe gazing at the canal? Standing in their back gardens, feeling the grass under their feet, wondering when all of this will end? A small bird looks at me, shakes its head and flutters to a tree.

Ireland's first case of Covid-19 was confirmed by the Health Protection Surveillance Centre on 29 February 2020.[5] The following day, a secondary school in the east of the country closed for two weeks after it confirmed that a male student had the virus. This unfortunate young man had just returned from an at-risk area of northern Italy. In truth, the virus had probably arrived in Ireland much earlier than this: he was simply the first documented case.

This marked the start of the first wave of the virus in Ireland. Stringent public health restrictions were soon imposed. By May 2020 there were moves towards relaxing the measures, but cases increased in August, especially in Kildare, Laois and Offaly. New restrictions were introduced in September 2020 to cope with a second wave. In early December 2020 measures were eased again, but a third wave emerged before the end of the month.

Today, in February 2021, it is clearer than ever that our hyper-connected world might have been designed for the spread of Covid-19. Extensive transmission was inevitable. Once the virus declared itself, efforts at containment, insofar as this was possible, required a careful combination of public health measures, political determination and psychological awareness. While medical interventions were always going to be key, they rarely achieve their goals without firm political support and an awareness that unhelpful psychological reactions can lead to hysteria, disengagement and nihilism.[6] This just makes everything worse.

A wise teacher once told me that humans have two fundamental responses to threat: panic and complacency.

Neither response is helpful and both were evident in early 2020, albeit about two different kinds of threat: panic about Covid-19 and complacency about other, apparently less dramatic problems, including climate change. My teacher overstated her point so that I would remember it—and, to her credit, I do, some 34 years later. Panic and complacency are everywhere.

One year on from Ireland's first case of Covid-19, some might argue that initial panic about the infection was more than justified. Much has changed, however, over the course of that year. The virus, still mysterious in some ways, has become familiar in others.

Inevitably, medical advice has shifted considerably, and improved. The World Health Organization (WHO) initially advised that people with no respiratory symptoms, such as cough, did not need to wear face-masks. Masks were recommended for people with symptoms of Covid-19 and people caring for those with symptoms, such as cough and fever. This included healthcare workers and people who were minding someone at home or in a healthcare facility. Initially, the WHO saw no reason why people outside these categories should wear masks.

This advice changed over time, as new facts emerged. Face-coverings became ubiquitous and will not disappear for some time to come, if ever. Other early advice stood the test of time: hygiene and targeted isolation remain effective measures to reduce transmission.

Compared to other viruses, the mortality rate with Covid-19 remains relatively low. Approximately 2 per cent of cases result in death. The mortality rate with Severe Acute Respiratory Syndrome (SARS) was approximately 10 per cent. Of course, high-level statistics are no consolation if you or a family member are in the 2 per cent of those with the virus who might die, as the pandemic showed.

While the savage onslaught of Covid-19 still feels raw and unprecedented, this experience is not new. Viruses, epidemics and pandemics have always exacted a terrible toll on humanity.[7] The global influenza pandemic that lasted from 1918 to 1920, also known as the Spanish 'flu, is, perhaps, the best-remembered pandemic of recent times, with at least 50 million deaths worldwide.[8]

Public health responses to these events have evolved over time, but psychological responses appear more constant: mixtures of complacency, appropriate anxiety, excessive anxiety and panic.[9] All of these reactions were evident in Ireland during the opening months of 2020, just as they were in all pandemics over the course of human history.

Seated here by the canal, one year into the current pandemic, I re-read William Wilde's 1856 summary of outbreaks, epidemics and pandemics in Irish history. Other people might be standing in their back gardens doing Tai Chi or meditating, but my head is buried in the 1851 census.[vi]

In the document, Wilde presents detailed information from multiple sources to sketch out grim histories that echo many of our experiences of Covid-19 today:

vi   I might have a problem.

Having found that, from the earliest period to which past chronicles refer down to the present time, Ireland has suffered sometimes alone, and sometimes in common with Great Britain and the rest of Europe, from various epidemic pestilences, we collected and tabulated the circumstances attending them in the table attached to these introductory remarks.

From an examination of this epitome of the most remarkable epidemic pestilences, as well as of the famines, epizootics, cosmical phenomena, and other circumstances, influencing, or supposed to influence mortality, we perceive that so far as the annals and records of the country afford information, Ireland has from the earliest period of its colonization to the present time been subjected to a series of dire calamities, affecting human life, arising either from causes originating within itself, or from its connexion with Great Britain and other parts of Europe.[10]

The causes of these unfortunate events, including pandemics, were many and varied, according to Wilde:

The literature of the times and the history of those early plagues, which devastated different parts of the world, show us that men usually endeavoured to account for such sudden outbursts of disease, either by the direct and miraculous interposition of Providence, or by some peculiar atmospheric condition, the manifestations of which were storms, hail, thunder, and lightning, unusual or sudden alterations of temperature, such as excessive heat, long continued drought, intense frost and snow, or great rains and inundations.

Occasionally 'signs and wonders', eclipses of the sun or moon, comets, and certain prodigies and supernatural appearances in the heavens, are said to have been the forerunners of these disasters, affecting the animal or the vegetable world; and during the middle ages of the Christian era, the failure of crops, a murrain among cattle, or an epidemic affecting the human family, were often considered as punishments from heaven, for sacrilege or other crimes of that nature.

Wilde showed a shrewd understanding of the epidemiology and spread of infectious diseases—an understanding that is just as relevant to Covid-19 as it was in ancient Ireland:

Many of the plagues from which this country suffered were continuations of those great waves of pestilence which had already passed (according to the general course of plagues) from the East, over the European continent, frequently carried along the track of human intercourse, by commercial dealings, or borne onward by hostile navies or invading armies; but others were more localised, were of domestic growth, and had their birth, and expended themselves within the circuit of this island—seldom spreading beyond its limits.

A century and a half later, Covid-19 was, in one sense, carried 'from the East, over the European continent', to

Ireland via Italy, 'along the track of human intercourse', as Wilde puts it. But while Wilde's words ring true to an eerie degree today, this simple account underestimates the extent to which a great many of us co-created the Covid-19 pandemic.

When we consider not only the emergence of the virus but also its transmission and transformation into a global pandemic, other factors emerge: the way we unbalance our environment with urbanisation, industrial animal-farming and ceaseless global travel; the way we create societies of such inequity that the health of millions of people suffers and many lack access to sanitation and basic medicines, let alone vaccines; and the way we reliably fail to coordinate early responses to all kinds of events, from floods to political instability, from climate change to pandemics.

When it comes to the causes of the Covid-19 *pandemic*, we are all in this together.

MARCH 2021

The month of March pays homage to Mars, the Roman god of war and father of Romulus and Remus. In Shakespeare's Julius Caesar, *a soothsayer warned the emperor to 'beware the ides of March'. Caesar dismissed the gloomy prognosticator: 'He is a dreamer; let us leave him'. Caesar was unwise: he was assassinated on the fifteenth of the month. March was once considered the first month of the year and it heralds the arrival of spring. Charles Dickens captured the contradictions of the month in*

Great Expectations: *'It was one of those March days when the sun shines hot and the wind blows cold: when it is summer in the light, and winter in the shade'.*

February melts into March. On 11 March 2021, it is precisely one year since the WHO classified the Covid-19 outbreak as a pandemic. While most people who contract the virus have a relatively mild, self-limiting illness, it can prove fatal, especially among those with pre-existing illness or limited access to healthcare. Old injustices are writ large. One year ago, in March 2020, the outbreak seemed to slip out of control, especially among the poor.

Viruses and pandemics expose the inequities of human society as much as they demonstrate nature's limitless ability to generate new infections. Exploring early Irish literature, Wilde found particularly 'striking' accounts of 'the first and second outbreaks of the *Blefed*, or *Buidhe Connail*—the great Yellow Plague, which devastated Ireland in the sixth and seventh centuries', especially among the poor.[11] He went on to present his detailed 'Table of Cosmical Phenomena, Epizootics, Famines, and Pestilences in Ireland', starting in 'the Pagan or Pre-Christian Period' and drawn, in large part, from sources such as the *Annals of the Four Masters*, chronicles of medieval Irish history compiled in the 1630s.

Wilde's first entry in the Table recounts the deaths of 5,000 men and 4,000 women in one week in 'the place now called Tallaght, near Dublin', in 'the year of the world

2820, according to the long chronology of the Septuagint' (approximately 2680 BC).[12] Their deaths were attributed to 'some sudden epidemic' which was 'the first recorded pestilence in Ireland'. Unlike Covid-19, the precise nature of this outbreak is still obscure and will likely remain so forever.

I cannot help noticing that this early 'pestilence' took place in Tallaght, where I now work and where Tallaght University Hospital dealt with Covid-19 patients right throughout the current pandemic. There is historical symmetry here—and enormous progress. I have never seen such selfless dedication as I saw among our hospital staff during the darkest days of Covid-19. My colleagues did not hesitate for a second: they donned their PPE and stepped (carefully) towards the risk when they needed to, rather than away from it. I have never felt so humbled.

Wilde continues his 1856 list with an astonishing catalogue of epidemics, plagues, cosmic events and desperately unfortunate occurrences to beset Ireland over the centuries, some of dubious veracity. The *Annals of Innisfallen* record '(*Bolgach*) smallpox amongst the people' in AD 569.[13] Wilde is sceptical: 'This is the first notice of this disease in the Irish annals, and one of the earliest references thereto in any European authority. As it is not, however, verified in any other annal, the epidemic alluded to was probably the leprosy, then epidemic.'

The *Annals of Boyle* record 'a great pestilence (*mortalitas magna*), that is the *Buidhe Chonnaill*' in the (ominous) year of 666.[14] 'Diarmaid and Blathmac, the two Kings of Ireland, died, as did Fechin of Fore, and many others thereof'.[vii]

In 675 'there reigned a kind of great leprosie in Ireland this year, called the Pox, in Irish, *Bolgagh*'. This, according to Wilde, 'evidently was the small-pox, of which many distinguished persons died'.

Mysteries and tragedies abound. In 678 'Lough Neagh was turned into blood'. The following year saw 'universal pestilence', as 'England and Ireland were ravaged by it in 679; and in 680, during July, August and September, Rome was laid waste'. The year 695 saw 'the cattle pestilence'.[15] There was 'a great cow mortality' in 707. In 742 there was both 'the *Bolgach*—small-pox' and 'dragons seen in the sky'.[16] In 814 there was 'a great disease' and 'heavy sickness (*Tromghalar*)'.[17]

Some entries in Wilde's Table are deeply obscure. In 847, 'Felym MacCriowhayn was overtaken by a great flux of the belly'. No further explanation is offered or, indeed, desired.[viii]

There has always been an element of the mysterious and the unknowable about sudden illnesses, plagues and

vii   Féichín was a seventh-century Irish saint. He founded a Christian
      monastery in Fore, Co. Westmeath. Today, the 'Seven Wonders
      of Fore' include a monastery in a bog, a mill without a race, water
      that flows uphill, a tree that won't burn, water that won't boil, an
      anchorite in a stone (a hermit's cell) and a lintel stone raised by St
      Fechin's prayers. Fore is worth a visit. The water really flows uphill.
      I've seen it.
viii 'Flux of the belly' is not an established medical diagnosis, but it
      sounds desperately unpleasant.

epidemics. This is evident in Wilde's accounts of historical outbreaks, and was also apparent when Covid-19 appeared in 2020. The arrival of the virus had been heralded for several weeks, as the crisis deepened in Italy, but the first Irish case still felt like a shock.

This month, in early March 2021, Minister for Finance Paschal Donohoe reflects on 'The Pandemic: One Year On' in a speech to the Economic and Social Research Institute. The Minister comments especially on the emotionally arresting nature of the early stages of the outbreak:

> The changes we have all seen over the past year have been profound. So many moments of that year will be indelibly etched into my memory. The moment I heard of this virus. The moment the scale of potential harm and death became clear […] Just twelve months ago, no one would have believed the year we were about to endure.[18]

Consistent with his brief, the Minister closes his remarks with a positive message:

> To conclude, vaccination is now being rolled out across the country and the beginning of the end is, hopefully, now in sight. Many of our youngest citizens returned to school earlier this week and, all going to plan, more will return in mid-March. The challenges are great, but we have achieved much and, in our national efforts to prevail over this disease, we will achieve more.

The Minister is right. With Covid-19 we have achieved far more than with any other outbreak in history: better treatment for the seriously ill, better vaccines (at least in rich countries) and better understanding of how the infection is transmitted.

Some old patterns remain, however, and would be familiar to Wilde, were he alive today. While the early spread of Covid-19 emphasised the interconnectedness of the modern world, as the virus clearly tracked flight paths from China and Italy, infections have always spread between countries. This is not new. Wilde draws an example from the *Annals of Ulster*, which record 'a great Leprosy (*Clamthruscad mor*, scaly leprosy or mange) and running of blood (*Ruith fola*, dysentery) upon the Gentiles of Dublin' in 950:

> These two notices would appear to apply to Syphilis, (and if so, to fix the introduction of it into Ireland), and the circumstances of the period tend to favour that idea. For some years before, there had been several Danish invasions, and immediately preceding the year 950 the Danes plundered a great part of Leinster, and took many captives—in one instance 'upwards of three thousand persons', so that the accession and spread of venereal affections is likely to have occurred at the time referred to.[19]

Wilde clearly blames Danish invaders for bringing syphilis to Ireland and spreading it around, not the native Irish. While this convenient allegation remains unproven, he does present compelling evidence that early Irish history was replete with epidemic illnesses (often said to come from abroad), unlikely misfortunes (frequently involving the unexpected appearance of blood) and bizarre cosmic occurrences (many of which strain credulity). It is stirring, disturbing stuff.[ix]

At the end of his 'Table of Cosmical Phenomena, Epizootics, Famines, and Pestilences in Ireland', Wilde provides yet more details about certain events, especially those connected with blood. He recounts several occasions when 'Lough Neagh was turned into blood' (in 649 and 679, for example); the time 'a shower of honey, a shower of silver, and a shower of blood fell in Ireland' (683); and the appearance of 'a shower of pure silver, a shower of wheat, and a shower of honey' at Inishowen between 759 and 763.[20]

Wilde's accounts of illnesses, in particular, take on added significance today, more than a year after Ireland's first case of Covid-19 and in the light of the global devastation wrought by this pandemic. How bad did similar pandemics get in the past? Was anything ever worse than Covid-19?

Yes, things got much worse than this in the past. The 'Black Death' or bubonic plague raged in Ireland from 1348 to 1350, and it is likely that between a quarter and a third of the population died during the first outbreak.[21] Thankfully, Covid-19 does not come close to this death toll.

ix   Wilde sometimes mixes folklore with science, rumours with reliable
      reports. His writings benefit hugely as a result, even if the truth gets a
      little blurry from time to time.

There were several more epidemics of plague, which only declined across Europe in the mid-seventeenth century, at which point typhus and dysentery became the chief threats. Smallpox, too, was a major cause of death in eighteenth-century Ireland. An epidemic of typhus developed between 1816 and 1819, and was followed by cholera in the 1830s.

Wilde describes an earlier outbreak of typhus, in 1225, based on the *Annals of the Four Masters*. This episode demonstrates clear links between social conditions, poverty, illness and death, not unlike the distribution of mortality from Covid-19 today:

> 'An oppressive malady (*Teidhm diofhulaing*, irresistible pestilence) raged in the province of Connaught at this time [1225]; it was a heavy, burning sickness (*Treabhlaid Tromteasaiglithi*), which left the large towns desolate, without a single survivor'. This hot, heavy, death sickness, not sudden as the *tamh*, was probably our Irish typhus, which succeeded to the war and famine which desolated large portions of Ireland at this period; so that 'woeful was the misfortune which God permitted to fall upon the best province in Ireland at that time, for the young warriors did not spare each other, but preyed and plundered each other to the utmost of their power. Women and children, the feeble, and the lowly poor, perished by cold and famine in this war'.[22]

This link between illness and social conditions, so evident with Covid-19, was also apparent during the Great

Irish Famine of 1845 to 1849. These years saw epidemics of typhus, cholera, dysentery and smallpox, as well as 'mental disease', which 'bore its part in the list of calamities, upon which it is our duty to report', according to Wilde.[23] 'The receptions into Lunatic Asylums ... greatly increased and the deaths from insanity [became] greater from 1847 to 1850' as part 'of that great calamity which befell this country during the years of famine and pestilence'.

The nineteenth century was the asylum-building era in Ireland, when large public institutions for the mentally ill were erected across the country.[24] The new asylums were immediately overcrowded, fuelling fevered speculation that the rate of mental illness was increasing uncontrollably in Ireland (and elsewhere). It is now clear that Ireland had an epidemic of mental hospitals rather than an epidemic of mental illness, but at the time the panic was slow to subside, fuelled by the ever-expanding institutions, ill-advised mental health legislation and alarmist reports in professional and popular media. In addition, frequent epidemics provided a vocabulary of infection that was often applied to mental illness, albeit without cause.

Against this background, the early twentieth century saw the most dramatic pandemic of recent history, the global influenza pandemic or 'Spanish 'flu' that killed at least 50 million people worldwide between the spring of 1918 and the winter of 1919.[25] In Ireland the 'flu infected almost 800,000 people and more than 20,000 died.[26] The pandemic had enormous effects across Irish society. The large, overcrowded asylums were hit especially hard: a fifth of all patients in Belfast asylum died of the 'flu, and one patient in every seven in the asylums in Kilkenny, Castlebar, Maryborough and Armagh fell victim.[27]

Tuberculosis was another persistent problem in Ireland throughout much of the twentieth century, becoming the leading cause of death among Irish children in the 1930s.[28] It, too, had an especially powerful impact in the mental hospitals. The tuberculosis epidemic did not end until the late 1950s as a result of testing, vaccination and effective antibiotics.

The advent of Covid-19 in early 2020 prompted media comparisons of the new coronavirus virus not only with the Spanish 'flu and tuberculosis but also with HIV/AIDS in the 1980s, severe acute respiratory syndrome in 2003 (SARS, which caused no deaths in Ireland) and the influenza pandemic of 2009 ('swine 'flu', which led to 27 deaths in Ireland).[29] Such comparisons are interesting and useful provided that they are accompanied by an awareness that the medical, social, political and economic circumstances of each outbreak can be quite different.[30] As a result, each epidemic and pandemic is, in certain ways, unique.

Certainly, Covid-19 *feels* unparalleled to me, but that is likely because I am living through it. Logically, I know that it is not unprecedented.

As Wilde demonstrates, human history is a catalogue of epidemics, disasters and misfortunes, but each generation *feels* that its experiences are unprecedented, despite the fact that virtually everything that happens today has happened before, probably several times. One of the key differences with Covid-19 is, perhaps, that this is the first pandemic in over a century that has brought rich countries, such as Ireland, to their knees. As a result, it feels new and unprecedented, even if it is not.

Another difference between the current outbreak and those of the past is the enhanced role played by global networks of scientists, doctors and health officials in shaping governmental responses this time round. As early as March 2020, Will Hutton commented in *The Observer* that members of 'a global scientific community' were 'talking to each other even if national leaders are not':

> A reliable test was established within days as Covid-19's gene sequence was fast decoded. Vaccine prototypes exist and will soon be trialled on humans. Antiviral treatments are already being clinically trialled. There is an emerging consensus about the risks of infection, the mortality rate and the effectiveness of varying containment strategies. This can and will be beaten.[31]

Later in 2020, the arrival of vaccines was a game-changer. As March 2021 ends and we grind into our second year of Covid-19, it is the thought of vaccination that keeps many people going, keeps our hopes afloat. As someone who was privileged enough to be vaccinated early—privileged, indeed, to be vaccinated at all—I can attest to the brightness that it brought to a very dark period.

The arrival of the pandemic—in effect, a plague—is a fierce reminder of one of our darker human destinies: infection, illness, death. A pandemic is elemental. The threat is everywhere and invisible. The threat is other people—our worst fears realised. Our usual sources of support are now reservoirs of risk. We are told to reach out but cannot get too close.

Wilde had a keen understanding of human suffering. He rooted his 1856 census report in both statistics and stories. Numbers tell us a lot, but they do not tell us everything. History has rhythm and melody. Pandemics require both and transcend both.

At some level, we recognise Covid-19 as the drumbeat of deep time. *Abyssus abyssum invocat*: deep calls to deep, suffering to suffering, pandemic to pandemic.[x]

Covid-19 challenges us medically and morally, revealing our fragility, stretching our civility, invoking a generosity that is only seen in disasters. Our own suffering and that of others prompts many responses: to save oneself, to help other people, to wonder about the meaning of it all. *Natura nihil frustra facit*: nature does nothing in vain.[xi]

But why this? Why now? Why us? Are we being punished?

We torment ourselves when we search for meaning in nature. Nature eludes meaning. We can search for meaning in our response to nature and natural phenomena: people,

---

x   Everything sounds better in Latin.
xi   Seriously.

trees, viruses. But nature is without meaning in itself. That is its majesty.

APRIL 2021

'April' is the Roman name for the fourth month of the year. The word comes from the verb aperire, *which means 'to open', because trees and plants traditionally 'open' around now. To return to Shakespeare, in Sonnet 98: 'April, dressed in all his trim, hath put a spirit of youth in everything'. Poet William Cowper in the eighteenth century had a more cautious take on the month: 'It is a sort of April-weather life that we lead in this world. A little sunshine is generally the prelude to a storm.'*

Infections cause extraordinary pain and loss at all times, not just during pandemics. William Wilde's life was touched by darkness in 1867, when his beloved 9-year-old daughter Isola died, most likely of an infection. The effect on Wilde was sudden, immediate and profound.

Wilde had a complex personal life, resulting in many children. Born in Castlerea, Co. Roscommon, in March 1815, he studied medicine in Dublin and became a Licentiate of the Royal College of Surgeons in 1837. He married Jane Francesca ('Speranza') in 1851, but by that point already had three children: Henry, Emily and Mary, born in 1838, 1847 and 1849 respectively. Henry later assisted Wilde in his practice. Emily and Mary died tragically in 1871, after their dresses caught fire at a Hallowe'en party.

Following marriage, Wilde and Jane had three children: William, Oscar and Isola, born in 1852, 1854 and 1857 respectively. William became a journalist and poet. Oscar was a celebrated playwright. Isola, the youngest, was a notably chirpy, happy child, whom Wilde described as 'embodied sunshine'.[32]

Nine-year-old Isola died suddenly in the spring of 1867, owing to 'a sudden effusion on the brain', according to her mother. The most likely cause was meningitis, an acute inflammation of the membranes of the brain and spinal cord, usually attributable to an infection. Viruses, bacteria and other micro-organisms can all trigger meningitis. One of these was likely responsible for Isola's tragic death.

Wilde was distraught. A decade earlier, he had carefully documented the impact of infections in Ireland over several centuries, in his 1856 report on the 1851 census. Now, abruptly, the loss of his own daughter underlined the heartless injustice of infective illnesses, the cruel indifference of nature to the fate of man.

Half a century later, the Spanish 'flu pandemic would bring further sweeping losses in Ireland, as another infection swept the world, killing millions and leaving countless more bereaved. A century after that, Covid-19 emerged in China during the last week of December 2019. The pattern is as inevitable as it is shocking every time: infection, illness, death. Repeat *ad infinitum*.

As was the case in 1918 and in previous outbreaks recounted by Wilde, Covid-19 presented two immediate challenges to the world: the first was the illness caused by the virus itself and the second was the panic that it triggered around the globe.[33] The ubiquity of speculative and false information about Covid-19 presented particular problems for public understanding and rational management of the outbreak.[34] Such problems were not new. Exaggerations, rumours, myths and falsehoods abounded during the Spanish 'flu, causing confusion, distress and a great deal of panic.[35] A century later, social media amplified this issue and led to extraordinary misinformation and anxiety about Covid-19.

In February 2020, the WHO recognised this problem and took specific steps to stop inaccuracies and conspiracy theories from spreading across social and conventional media.[36] Reputable medical journals made reliable information available for health professionals.[37] These steps remain important. The experience of the Spanish 'flu clearly demonstrates the power of myths and the requirement for calm, factual information to counteract unhelpful panic.

Another lesson from the Spanish 'flu and earlier outbreaks is that infectious illnesses have profound psychological effects in addition to physical ones, as Wilde recognised only too well. Historian Ida Milne writes about the emotional effects of the Spanish 'flu, exploring the losses that people suffered and psychological traumas that lasted in many cases for a lifetime.[38] It is important to recognise these long-term psychological effects during all phases of the Covid-19 pandemic (even after it ends) and to offer psychological interventions to those who need them.[39]

Regrettably and inevitably, some of the public health measures required to control transmission of Covid-19, such as isolation and quarantine, can have negative effects on psychological well-being. While these strategies are effective for limiting the spread of infection, measures such as quarantine are also associated with specific stressors, such as fears of infection, frustration, boredom and problems stemming from inadequate supplies and insufficient information.[40] After quarantine, there can be concerns about finances and stigma, among other matters. These negative effects can be ameliorated by terminating quarantine as soon as possible, providing adequate information and supplies, reducing boredom and improving communication. These tasks are not easy, especially during a health emergency, but they are essential.

As was the case with the Spanish 'flu, many children's lives were deeply disrupted by Covid-19. The problems are particularly acute in children who were largely confined to home owing to school closures, family illness or physical distancing. In this setting, it was important that children were guided about on-line learning but not overburdened with work; that parents worked together with schools to ensure healthy lifestyles; and that good diet, personal hygiene and sleep habits were encouraged.[41] It is still useful for parents to have direct conversations with children about the outbreak, in order to alleviate persistent anxieties. The truth is a help, not a hindrance, even for younger children. They generally understand far more than we give them credit for.

One of the greatest psychological challenges of any pro-longed pandemic is learning to live with uncertainty not only about the virus but also about the evolving science that informs governmental and societal responses. Simon Jenkins summarised the dilemma neatly in *The Guardian* in April 2020, when he pointed out that the world was 'not divided between "the science" and other mortals':

> Scientists are like the rest of us. They form assumptions and grasp at evidence to validate them. They are optimists or pessimists, by nature risk-taking or cautious. My wife and I share inputs, hear the same news and read the same papers. But I am an optimist and she is a pessimist. I think we could have stuck to the Swedish model. I think the crisis will be over in three weeks. She believes it will last months. It is not much comfort that we both have scientists on our side.[42]

There is also protracted uncertainty about the outbreak's long-term effect on our societies and our way of life.[43] The epidemics during the Great Irish Famine and the Spanish 'flu had profound effects on Irish society. In this context it was important, from the start of Covid-19, to find time to reflect on our own thoughts and emotions about such uncertainty, to care for our physical health and to follow the mental health guidance provided by the WHO, among others.[44]

One of the other lessons from past epidemics and pan-demics is that everyone does not suffer equally: the poor were disproportionately affected by the epidemics of the Great Irish Famine, and people with mental illness were

31

especially vulnerable to the Spanish 'flu. One of the reasons for the latter was that so many of the mentally ill were confined in large, unhygienic mental hospitals through which 'flu spread at high speed. Today, mental health care is, for the most part, based in the community, but people with mental illness are still at increased risk of Covid-19.[45]

This injustice is neither new nor limited to infectious illnesses. Even prior to Covid-19, it was known that people with mental illness have a lower life expectancy and poorer physical health than the general population.[46] This places them at particularly increased risk in a pandemic, especially for community transmission of the virus. This underlines the importance of continued multi-disciplinary mental health care during the outbreak, despite the inevitable difficulties involved in delivering such care. The harder it is, the more it matters.

All of these health and social care interventions require broad-based community support in order to work. In March 2020, the WHO director-general emphasised the need for 'solidarity' in the face of Covid-19:

> There's still a lot we don't know, but every day we're learning more, and we're working around the clock to fill in the gaps in our knowledge. Ultimately, how deadly this virus will be depends not only on the virus itself, but on how we respond to it. This is a serious disease. It is not deadly to most people, but it can kill. We're all responsible for reducing our own risk of infection, and if we're infected, for reducing our risk of infecting others. There's something all of us can do to

protect vulnerable people in our communities. That's why we keep talking about solidarity. This is not just a threat for individual people, or individual countries. We're all in this together, and we can only save lives together.[47]

The WHO's idea that 'We're all in this together' came under serious pressure over the following year, as the pandemic's trajectory confirmed that healthcare is not delivered in a vacuum: containing the infection had as much to do with politics as it had to do with medicine. Viruses spread quickly in countries that are poor and lack strong, democratic governments with the support and confidence required to take unpopular decisions. For Covid-19, this was especially true in relation to issues such as quarantine, isolation, healthcare and vaccination.

Around the world, the distribution of diseases, deaths and cures has always been intensely political.[48] Poverty, inequality and politics inevitably matter deeply, as rich countries are better placed to contain outbreaks: better sanitation, better nutrition, better healthcare. The picture with Covid-19 was very different in poor countries, where most people who died of the virus died, in truth, of a toxic combination of poverty, inequality and infection.

In April 2020 Michael D. Higgins, President of Ireland, addressed this issue at the African–European Parliamentarians Initiative (AEPI) web-conference:

In Ireland we may be coming out of some of our worst experience through, really, the cooperation of the public, really respecting the advice of washing our hands, having an etiquette in relation to sneezing, social distancing, but I know very well that such advice is going to be so difficult in Africa, where you have overcrowding and in the periphery of cities where clean water is not available and where, as well as that, the idea of social isolating is simply impossible.

[...] We must respond to all of these conditions by realising the particularities of the African situation and we must do so, this time, in a way that will allow African agency, perhaps using African communities to develop the capacities, or strengthen the capacities where they are there, to deal with their own needs [...] If we are to learn from this crisis it should be that we shift the emphasis from armaments and from the debt we are encouraging in the world, to providing universal basic services.

I think, too, this is a great opportunity for Europe. Europe has had a legacy in Africa that it would like to forget, but which Africans have not forgotten. And I think now is an opportunity to make a new beginning and not only to respond to Covid-19 but also to respond to those structural imbalances that are there: unfair trade and then there is, of course, the burden of debt.[49]

Again, this story is not new. In 2019, months before Ireland's first case of Covid-19, President Higgins spoke about the Spanish 'flu in a speech titled 'The Great Flu of 1918–1919: Why Remember? Why Forget?':

Just over one hundred years ago, as the First World War was drawing to a fitful close, an influenza virus, unlike any before or since, swept across the world, felling soldiers and civilians alike.

The global death toll was inconceivable: according to the most recent estimates, between 50 million and 100 million people worldwide perished in the three pandemic waves between the spring of 1918 and the winter of 1919, making it one of the deadliest natural disasters in human history [...]

As with other 20th-century epidemics and pandemics, such as HIV/AIDS, Africans and Asians suffered proportionately more than Europeans and North Americans. Thus, while the average case mortality in what we term the developed world was about 2%, in India, where 18.5 million perished, it was 6%, and in Egypt, where 138,000 died, it was 10%. In isolated regions in which populations had no immunity to flu, the impact was truly astonishing: in Western Samoa, for example, a quarter of the population died, while in Alaska some entire Inuit communities died as a result.[50]

Today, at the end of April 2021, over a year since the Covid-19 pandemic was declared, infections and deaths are again unevenly distributed around the world. It was always thus.

The solutions remain, in large part, political: enhanced support and debt relief for poor countries, increased emphasis on public health, more transparent decision-making about scarce resources (such as vaccines), and explicit acknowledgement of the role of social and economic factors in physical and mental health. President Higgins is right: if 'structural imbalances' lie at the heart of the problem, correcting these 'imbalances' must lie at the heart of the solution.

Change requires political will. Rudolf Virchow, the great nineteenth-century German pathologist, anthropologist and politician, commented that 'medicine is a social science, and politics is nothing but medicine on a large scale'. Covid-19 proves him right—yet again.

With this in mind, it is easy to despair. If deep-rooted social injustice fuels the pandemic, can we ever hope to see the end of Covid-19? Will the world ever be the same? Should it ever be the same? What should we do next?

It is tempting to argue that a global crisis presents a unique opportunity for global improvement and renewal. But it is equally possible to argue the opposite: that a global crisis shifts attention and resources away from making the world a better place, delays human progress and expands the gap between rich and poor, as Covid-19 has done.

How can poor countries build back better, if they can barely build back at all?

MAY 2021

May is named for the Greek goddess Maia, daughter of Atlas and Pleione, and mother of Hermes. Maia is synonymous with growth. May is a month of blossoming. In Finn, Son of Cumhal, *Lady Gregory sings its praises: 'The month of May is the pleasant time; its face is beautiful; the blackbird sings his full song, the living wood is his holding, the cuckoos are singing and ever singing; there is a welcome before the brightness of the summer'.*

I struggle to stay in touch with the seasons, but even I cannot deny an early summer: the sun is beaming, the air is light and there is a brightness, a sweetness, a freedom in the ether.

Living and working in Dublin city, I often fail to notice when autumn turns to winter, spring to summer. It occasionally occurs to me that it is raining more than usual, or that the weather feels warmer, but the overarching pattern, the rhythm, is lost on me. I rush about the city, insensible to the turning of the seasons. I might as well be on Mercury.[xii]

Occasionally, I stop in my tracks, momentarily confused. If I cycle to work, I sometimes spot rabbits and their young in a park.[xiii] These catch my attention. I imagine they have seasonal significance, but I quickly move on.[xiv]

Christmas reminds me that it is winter, a fact that might otherwise escape me. If I am honest, only the most blatant reminders of the seasons impinge. Asked randomly what season it is, I would need to consult a calendar.

This was not the case with William Wilde, who was fiercely attuned to the rhythms of nature. In 1867 he wrote about the seasonal flora of his beloved west of Ireland in

xii Technically, Mercury does not have seasons.
xiii Baby rabbits are called 'kittens', it seems.
xiv They do indeed have seasonal significance: peak breeding time is
     April to June.

his book *Lough Corrib, its Shores and Islands: with Notices of Lough Mask:*

> Of the various heaths and ferns in Connemara we have not now time or space to speak; but there is one plant that has given such a tone to the landscape, that we cannot refrain from a passing notice of it—the *Narthicium*, or Bog Asphodel, that abounds everywhere throughout Connemara, and forms the chief plant upon the surface of our great mosses, and the long white roots of which compose the principal portion of the upper layer of turf. It grows up everywhere; and the moment man's efforts at cultivation cease, it reasserts its rights, and spreads with immense rapidity.
>
> In spring, its slender, bent-like leaves of bluish-green freshen the surface; in summer its yellow blossoms give a rich warm tint to the landscape; and in autumn, when it bears a brownish-red seed, and the tops of its leaves turn crimson, it presents us with another colour, equally rich and impressive; while it also feeds hundreds of black cattle.[51]

Wilde writes about autumn a good deal. He describes hills 'brown with bog, and dappled with the grey bare rocks that rise towards their summits, or margin the streams that course down their rugged sides, and in autumn are purple with occasional stripes of heather, which the continuous waterflow along their sides has permitted to enjoy a partial inflorescence'.[52]

Elsewhere, 'the rugged scarped sides of the mountains overhanging Maam', when 'lighted by autumn sunsets playing on the russet tints of the projecting crags, produce flecks of a burnished coppery hue of surpassing loveliness'.[53] It is stirring, seasonal stuff.

As ever, Wilde mixes facts and observations with myths and stories to paint a deeper, fuller, truer picture. He visits a castle that is 'often seen, it is said, "afire" on summer nights, when the fairies, after their game of hurling, hold their banquets there'.[54] He recounts the fairies' summer parties with utmost gravity, using the same tone that he employs in the census reports when he discusses Lough Neagh turning 'into blood' in the seventh century, or showers of silver, wheat and honey falling at Inishowen during the eighth.[55] These are all events of note, each as true as the next, each harbouring meaning of one sort or other, even as literal and metaphorical truths sometimes merge.

It is Wilde's closeness to nature that strikes me the most, in my somewhat alienated urban life. Distance from the seasons troubles me.

When public health restrictions tightened during 2020 and many people spent more time at home, some reported heightened awareness of their surroundings, increased consciousness of their environments and deepened mindfulness of the seasons. The term 'long time' emerged, to describe endless days spent working in 'home offices', or waiting for Covid-19 tests and results, or self-isolating at home, or 'cocooning' away from the world. Usual rhythms, defined by work, family and friends, were replaced by the deadening rhythm of daily statistics about the pandemic. The effect on our minds was impoverishing and stark.

On 1 May 2020, Taoiseach Leo Varadkar spoke about the impact of the 'Covid-19 emergency' on our mental states:

> The last few weeks have changed and transformed our lives in so many different ways. I know it has been difficult— sometimes dispiriting. The frustration of having our lives restricted. The uncertainty about when things will get back to normal. The fear of the virus itself.
>
> As a nation our physical health has been attacked, our mental health eroded, our economy battered, and our society put to the ultimate test. Many people are lonely and enduring the pain of isolation. Many people are grieving in silence. Many have lost their jobs. Many fear losing their businesses and many have lost their lives.
>
> I know, for me, the worst part has been the daily text message at around 5.30 every evening with the latest number of notified deaths and newly diagnosed cases. I yearn for the day when it stops.[56]

Over a year later, as I write this diary in May 2021, the daily case numbers have not yet stopped. Our physical health is still attacked, our mental health remains under pressure, the economy is struggling, and our society remains in the midst of a prolonged test of character and endurance. We talk about Covid-19 constantly. It dominates our lives. Does anything else even exist anymore?

While there is plentiful discussion of the psychological effects of the pandemic on the population at large, there is less consideration of its physical impact on people who are not infected with the virus. What are the biological effects of staying at home, remaining within 5km of our dwellings and upending the patterns of our daily lives that—for better or worse—defined our existences before the pandemic?

At both the psychological and the biological level, early 2020 saw the usual routines of our lives replaced by breathless anticipation of daily statistics and anxiety about government announcements. We hung on every word from the taoiseach and our public health officials. Over those months, I gazed intently at the television screen each evening to see whether our chief medical officer was smiling. If he was, that would mean more to me than any statistics.

If there was ever a time to tune in to the seasons of the year, this was it. If the drumbeat of deep time was reflected in the pandemic, then the seasons provided an alternative drumbeat to keep us sane, one of the few rhythms of normal life unaffected by Covid-19. Nothing stops the spring.

But this enhanced sensibility was not to be, for many people—at least not for me and various others. Not only did my lifestyle leave me unmoored from seasonal shifts before the pandemic began but also my work schedule persisted and often intensified as the emergency deepened. Working from home was simply impossible, for the most part.

Like many healthcare workers, the most significant change was to activities *in* my workplace rather than outside it: radically changed patient profiles, new infection control practices in the hospital and at our clinics, a crash course on how to don and remove PPE, and ever-changing protocols for managing ever-changing risk. As knowledge evolved, so did work practices. All the parts were moving parts. Nothing stayed stable for long in the early months of the pandemic.

In other words, there was no 'long time' at home. No 'home office'. No prolonged periods of quietude during which to deepen awareness of the environment and start to notice seasonal shifts. Other people had very different experiences, often feeling trapped at home for weeks and months on end, longing to get out into the wider world. This was not my experience.

All told, I consider myself fortunate, for three reasons.

First, I still had work to go to. Unlike so many other people, I was still employed. That is always something for which to be grateful.

Second, having permission to leave home to go to work, even during deepest lockdown, was good for my psychological well-being. Activity helps, especially gainful activity. Work gives purpose, structure and—on a good day—meaning. Having most people work from home was essential to reduce transmission of the virus, but there were psychological benefits when one simply had to leave the house and go into work.

Third, leaving home when restrictions were at their tightest provided memories that are etched in my mind forever. Driving to work along deserted roads that were previously choked with traffic. Producing my 'essential worker' letter at the frequent Garda checkpoints. Waving at other motorists: we were few in number on the road, so a sense of camaraderie developed. I will never forget those mornings. Some days, I might have been driving on the moon, deserted and alone.

Today, in May 2021, over a year since the start of the pandemic, the physical situation has changed dramatically (fewer restrictions, more motorists), but the psychological freeze is slow to thaw. The virus lingers stubbornly, even as we vaccinate with vigour. There is a sense of mourning, mixed with hope.

What have we lost? We have lost so much. Many have died. More have suffered other losses: loss of health, loss of loved ones, loss of employment, loss of security, loss of peace of mind.

What did we lose as a collective, as a people? We lost the rhythms of daily life and many of the patterns of our worlds, all of which are slow to return. We lost our easy assumptions of invulnerability and our sense of security. These will be even slower.

Our world-view was turned on its head, as dramatic new narratives emerged about our lives and our surroundings. Our starting-point was not good: just as I missed the seasons of the year for the first forty-seven years of my life, society suffered from 'mythic deprivation' until Covid-19 arrived, according to Tobias Jones in *The Observer*:

There has been no belonging and thus no community, no heroes and no quests. Suddenly we have all the above. But it's not entirely like a film where the heroes would be the medics dying to save us [...] and the quest would be the global race to find a vaccine. They're just a part of this story. Heroism for the rest of us is much subtler and quieter: it's about restraint and retreat, solitude and stillness. And our quest is perhaps even harder: to discern the common good and look for enlightenment in this darkness.[57]

In the bleakest days of this pandemic, concepts such as 'enlightenment' seemed impossibly distant from our experiences. Even today, it remains difficult to draw anything good from Covid-19. With so much grieving and rebuilding to do, how can we even start?

Over a century and a half before the current pandemic, William Wilde understood that the search for 'enlightenment' following such events involves the careful collection of numbers, information and stories about our experiences. How else can we describe what happened and start to understand?

Thus, Wilde created his extraordinary 'Table of Cosmical Phenomena, Epizootics, Famines, and Pestilences in Ireland' in his 1856 census report, which remains so absorbing today in ways that Wilde could not have imagined.

Then, as now, statistics were both essential and imperfect ways to describe and explain human experience. Wilde understood that extensive statistical records for both Ireland and neighbouring countries were needed in order to present a clear picture of something as complex as a transnational pandemic. Many of the records were, he said, 'defective':

> We feel, however, that in this publication of the annals of disease and blight in one of the most distant islands of the West, we are setting an example which, if followed up, will eventuate in such a better understanding of the history of epidemics, as may lead to the discovery of the laws by which they are governed, and thus enable mankind to provide in some measure against their influence.[58]

Wilde was right: the limits of statistics, such as daily case numbers of Covid-19, should not blind us to their value. Numbers are always imperfect, but they are one way to quantify what is going on, identify who is suffering and figure out what helps.

But numbers never tell the whole story. That is a key lesson from Wilde's writings about illness and pandemics: statistics, though essential, are not enough.

Lough Neagh never turned into blood, but those who said that it did were trying to convey something important, so Wilde included it in his account. Showers of silver, wheat and honey never fell at Inishowen, but something happened that could only be described in such dramatic terms. Wilde listened.

We need to listen too. With Covid-19, both numbers and stories matter. They always do.

2. SUMMER 2021: COPING

'Medicine to produce health must examine disease; and music to create harmony must investigate discord.'

—*Plutarch*

This chapter moves from June to August 2021, as Covid-19 cases persist, vaccination continues and public health restrictions gradually relax. The long-term effects of this pandemic are not yet clear. Even the short-term impacts are still under debate, although certain facts are undeniable: more than four million people have died, including over 5,000 in Ireland. Around the world, millions more are ill, bereaved or chronically anxious. How do we come back from this? William Wilde, in his travels in the Mediterranean in 1837, saw illness, plague and the consequences of infection all around him. It is no surprise that he later focused on these themes in his 1856 report on the 1851 census and in his clinical work. It is even less surprising that Wilde's writings speak so eloquently to us today, in the era of Covid-19. Infection is eternal. These summer months see significant changes in Ireland as the pandemic generally eases, although there is continued anxiety, restriction and difficulty adjusting to a world that is both changed and familiar, pervaded by worry and—despite everything—filled with promise.

JUNE 2021

June is named after Juno, the Roman goddess of marriage. This month marks the official start of summer. Henry David Thoreau felt that June brings us closer to the land: 'It is dry, hazy June weather. We are more of the earth, farther from heaven these days.' Mark Twain agreed: 'It is better to be a young June-bug than an old bird of paradise'. Edgar Allan Poe found himself in touch with nature during the brief summer nights: 'At midnight, in the month of June, I stand beneath the mystic moon'. I dislike the heat in June, but who am I to question Thoreau, Twain and Poe? It is summer and there is a 'mystic moon' as I write these words. That is enough.

June 2021. We are more than a year into the Covid-19 pandemic. Vaccination is under way and more successful than anyone expected. Less than a year ago, scientists warned—reasonably—that a vaccine might take years to develop or might never appear at all. In the event, science moved faster than anyone dared to hope. Priority groups were vaccinated in early 2021. The challenge now is to distribute vaccines as quickly as possible to as many people as feasible. It is an enormous, urgent undertaking.

In the meantime, people continue to contract Covid-19. Today, 18 June 2021—to take a random example—the Health Protection Surveillance Centre is notified of 373 new cases.[1] There are fifty-four Covid-19 patients in hospital, of whom eighteen are in intensive care. Even so, Dr Tony Holohan, Chief Medical Officer at the Department of Health, has reason to be optimistic owing to the vaccination programme and widespread compliance with public health measures:

> We are now experiencing near elimination of Covid-19 in the vaccinated population. For the 50–65s who are in the process of receiving protection from full vaccination, incidence is dropping. Incidence is also reducing in most age groups, showing commendable compliance with public health measures as the vaccination programme is rolled out to more and more people.

Dr Holohan has good news for people who have received their vaccines:

> If you are fully vaccinated you can safely resume normal life—meeting other fully vaccinated people from up to two households indoors without masks or social distancing, and meeting unvaccinated people from one other household indoors and without masks. Those of us awaiting vaccination should continue to wash/sanitise hands regularly, manage contacts, avoid crowds, wear masks where appropriate and socialise outdoors.

This is a dramatic change from just six months ago, when cases were rising, vaccines were not available and restrictions were very tough. Professor Philip Nolan, chair of the National Public Health Emergency Team (NPHET) Irish Epidemiological Modelling Advisory Group, matches Holohan's optimism today:

> All indicators of the disease are improving nationally. In April/May incidence was stable at 400–500 cases a day— this has now reduced to a five-day average of 303. Hospital admissions have reduced from 103 to 57 in the past two weeks. If we can continue to weigh public health measures with vaccine uptake and continue to keep new variants, including Delta, at bay, then the risk profile of Covid-19 in Ireland will alter for the better.

So what now? If we get enough jabs in arms, will our old lives resume over the coming months? Or will the Delta variant prove craftier than its predecessors? Vaccination is astonishingly good at reducing the risk of serious illness and death, but it is not 100 per cent effective, especially for preventing infection. How will this shake out?

Exactly one year ago, on 18 June 2020, when the outlook was much more uncertain, Richard Horton, editor-in-chief of *The Lancet* medical journal, published a provocative book titled *The Covid-19 Catastrophe: What's Gone Wrong and How To Stop It Happening Again*.[2] Horton argued that we are living through a period of unique political, economic and social instability, not to mention ubiquitous anxiety, owing to Covid-19. He felt that the virus would be with us for a long time, but that a catastrophe like this can be a catalyst for political and social change. What might such change look like?

Horton argued that, as a result of the pandemic, policy-makers would pay more attention to social capital (the informal ties that bind societies together), governments would find improved means for co-ordination and leadership, societies would demand better social protection, medicine would change in myriad ways (including more emphasis on public health) and scientific research would speed up and integrate better into clinical care. For Horton, Covid-19 is not an event but the start of a new phase of human history.[i]

I think most people understand how Horton feels. This feels like a period of enormous change, maybe even revolution. Can life ever return to the way it was before the pandemic? Surely something like Covid-19 means that many things have changed forever—or does it?

One year after Horton's book, in June 2021, it is not yet clear whether he was right on all points. Or, more precisely, it is not yet clear to what extent Horton's predictions will be realised in time. The long-term effects of the pandemic are not yet apparent.

I certainly hope that many of the changes that Horton envisions come to pass, but I imagine they will take time.

---

i   Horton gave a humdinger of an interview to the *Financial Times*: A. Ahuja, 'We've had the biggest science policy failure in a generation', *Financial Times*, 25/26 April 2020.

Right now, the pandemic still rages and there is little evidence of enhanced global leadership or co-ordination. The divergence between rich and poor countries has grown more rather than less stark. The arrival of vaccines, which appeared after Horton's book, has widened that chasm.

On the plus side, and in line with Horton's predictions, there is plenty of rhetoric about building social capital, strengthening public health frameworks and accelerating scientific research, even if most of these areas have not yet improved in a lasting way. The arrival of vaccines is the most striking exception, as the new jabs reflect the best application of recent science to an immediate public health problem in the history of medicine.

It is the politics of vaccines that is letting us down, not the science. The global poor are simply not getting inoculated, while the global rich (like me) are. Maybe Horton is an optimist; maybe nothing will really change.

In a world of such injustice, in which millions die of Covid-19 and I am privileged to be vaccinated, I feel guilty listing the things that I miss during this stage of the pandemic: visiting my family, going to the cinema, travelling abroad, and not worrying about everything the moment I leave the house. Am I standing too close to someone? How many people are in this shop? Have I inadvertently broken the rules and made other people anxious?

I desperately miss foreign travel. I love to head away—the farther, the better. The more discombobulated I am when I arrive somewhere, the more I like it. Nothing compares to the sensation of foreignness, exoticism and disorientation that overwhelms me when I step off an airplane in India, China or Japan. In early 2020, just as the pandemic reached Ireland, I had numerous trips planned: London, Spain, Rome, Russia. All were scrapped when international travel stopped abruptly.

Was every one of these trips necessary? Possibly not, but I mourned their loss at the time—and I still do.

Some of this travel was for work: a teaching stint in Rome and conferences in London and Russia. The pandemic has shown that we can do a great deal of this kind of work from home, using technologies like Zoom, at much less cost to the environment. And therefore we should.

But we cannot do everything remotely. My planned trips to Rome and Russia included visits to hospitals and universities, as well as various other expeditions. Technology offers enormous opportunities to reach out, but there is nothing quite like being there. I travelled to Russia many years ago and I long to return. Connecting by Zoom simply does not compare to visiting a psychiatric hospital in Moscow or standing by the river in St Petersburg, freezing in the Russian night.

William Wilde loved to travel, especially in his younger years. Just after he gained his medical degree from the Royal College of Surgeons in Ireland in 1837, he was recommended for the position of medical attendant on a nine-month cruise in the Mediterranean with a recovering tubercular patient, Robert Meiklam, a wealthy Glasgow merchant with a 130-tonne yacht, the *Crusader*.

Wilde, who suffered from asthma, did not need to be asked twice:

Anxiety to see the world, coupled with the fact of my own health being then in a precarious state, induced me gladly to accept of this kind offer. At their suggestion, I undertook to collect information relative to the *climate* of the places we should visit, and also to keep a register of their temperature. At the solicitation of other friends, I made a daily note of those objects which struck me as interesting in the countries we visited.[3]

In 1840 Wilde published a two-volume account of his travels, with a wonderful title: *Narrative of a Voyage to Madeira, Teneriffe, and Along the Shores of the Mediterranean, Including a Visit to Algiers, Egypt, Palestine, Tyre, Rhodes, Telmessus, Cyprus, and Greece, with Observations on the Present State and Prospects of Egypt and Palestine, and on the Climate, Natural History, Antiquities, etc. of the Countries Visited.*[ii]

The *Crusader* set sail from England on 24 September 1837. The vessel 'slipt past the white cliffs of the Isle of Wight, to seek for her inmates in warmer climes that health which an English winter cannot afford'.[4] Wilde's sights were also set on knowledge, adventure and exploration, as well as better health.

---

ii   Book titles have diminished in ambition, length and majesty over the years. Sigh.

The first stop was 'Corunna' (now A Coruña), a city in north-west Spain. Wilde describes the local dress in detail. He writes that the women 'wear no bonnets, but the graceful mantilla of black silk, trimmed with velvet and edged with lace, is drawn half-way over the head'.[5] As for the men:

> The gentlemen citizens are all enveloped in the cloak, above which are just seen a pair of formidable moustaches; but I never could divest myself of the idea of their having the deadly, treacherous stiletto hidden in its dark folds. They seem partial to the brightest colours; scarlet trousers being a favourite piece of dress.[6]

In Portugal, Wilde was 'disappointed with the city of Lisbon; and much more so with its climate, which was to us very trying, owing to the great transition from heat in the sunshine to cold in the shade'.[7] He had a very different response to the island of Madeira, which was already an established health resort:

> Far be it from me to say that the climate of Madeira *can cure consumption* [tuberculosis]; but this I will say, that, independent of its acknowledged efficacy in chronic affections, it is one that will do more to ward off threatened diseases of the chest, or even to arrest them in their incipient stages, than any I am acquainted with. A dry, warm climate, with a healthy and equable state of the atmosphere, are, no doubt, the most powerful remedial agents we are acquainted with.[8]

Madeira more than made up for the travails of the voyage so far. As the travelling party moved along, Wilde kept himself busy recording everything he saw: weather, plants, people, towns. The city of Santa Cruz on Tenerife was 'clean' and had 'a good square, La Plaza de la Constituçion':

> The houses of this Spanish colony are large, well built, and in the Moorish style of the mother country, having courts in the centre, surrounded by galleries. In many of those are handsome fountains, playing to a great height, which render them cool and refreshing.[9]

The heat bothered Wilde, so he valued any relief from it. Notwithstanding this irritation, his spirit was unquenched, and he explored Tenerife with gusto:

> As I proceeded into the hills, I observed the *euphorbium canariensis* [the Canary Island spurge, a poisonous succulent shrub that looks like a cactus] growing to an immense size; it looks like so many great candelabra, and this similitude is increased from the quantity of juice exuding, which crusts over the stalks and rocks beneath, with a yellowish wax-like paste.
>
> Some idea may be formed of the virulence of the poison of this plant from the following circumstance. I made incisions in some of the plants, in order to allow the milky juice to exude, and laid the point of the penknife I had used for an *instant* on the tip of my tongue: almost immediately I felt an intense heat, dryness, and burning

sensation in the fauces, back of the throat, and gullet, and suffered so much from weakness, that I was scarcely able to crawl back to the town.

On examination, there was no redness or inflammation to be seen, and the symptoms gradually subsided in the course of three or four hours, leaving, however, a huskiness which lasted several days.[10]

That kind of adventure is one of the things I miss most during Covid-19: the unpredictability of travel abroad. There is much to explore in Ireland, but the exoticism of distant lands has a special allure. I might not be as adventurous as Wilde, tasting random plants by the roadside,[iii] but I still miss the strangeness of 'other' countries: sights, smells, tastes, adventures.[iv] In a world in which millions have died of Covid-19, this is a minor complaint, but it is something that has affected me since the start of the pandemic.

It is the 'unknowing' that attracts me and that I miss most deeply when I cannot travel to distant lands: being confused, getting lost, not knowing where I am going or how to get there—let alone how to return.[v]

Predictably, it was difficult to achieve this feeling within 5km of my home during deep lockdown. I had double

iii   Born to be Wilde.
iv   Born to be mild.
v   I write about this in considerable, possibly excessive, detail in Chapter 10 of my book *The Science of Happiness: The Six Principles of a Happy Life and the Seven Strategies for Achieving it* (Dublin: Gill Books, 2021).

espressos at every coffee-shop within the 78.54km^2 circle surrounding my house, but nothing compared to the two harsh shots of caffeine that I had in Dubai airport in 2019, so strong that I needed to rest for fifteen minutes just to calm the dizziness. I miss that.

Today, in June 2021, restrictions have eased considerably. Foreign travel is possible, but only under certain circumstances and with various requirements and restrictions. These regulations, Byzantine but necessary, have changed the fundamental nature of travel, at least for now. It is no longer possible to travel to Germany and suddenly decide to visit Poland or head to the Netherlands for a few days. That is a loss—not so much for the places we might miss, but for the sense of freedom and security in the world that such travel represented.

This kind of travel was a rite of passage for many young adults in rich, privileged countries like Ireland over past decades. If today's young people do not have these experiences now, will they have the opportunity again in the future? Or will their understanding of travel be permanently different, as their formative years are shaped not only by the pandemic and its disruption to education but also by the implicit message that the world is more dangerous than we thought? That travel is forever fraught with unknowable risk?

There are compelling arguments against thoughtless travel, based on climate impact and global inequity, but arguments based on ideas of infinite danger and anxiety are surely to be avoided. If we stay at home or travel differently in order to save the planet or increase global justice, that is one thing and is greatly to be desired. But if we stay at home out of fear, even after the pandemic is over, that is something else entirely, greatly to be avoided. The world is there to be saved, cherished, shared and explored, not feared.

Managing attitudes towards risk was always going to be a tricky part of our response to Covid-19. From the outset, it was clear that good communication and solidarity would be key. Early on, the Department of Health began daily media briefings. There were regular updates on the websites of the HSE and WHO. We all learned a new language: coronavirus, delay phase, mitigation, flattening the curve.[11]

The public health messages and this new terminology made perfect sense, especially in the early days of the pandemic. Someone knew what they were doing. We instinctively understood the need for social distance. Certain people needed to self-quarantine. Others had to self-isolate to protect family and friends. International travel essentially ceased. This all made sense. After all, there was a pandemic, of all things.

But while these messages and measures were entirely logical, their emotional impact was confusing. We were told that we were all in this together but needed to stay two metres apart. We had to care for the vulnerable but could not visit our mothers on Mothers' Day. And, if we were tested for Covid-19, we had to assume that the test was positive and self-isolate until we heard the result, even if we now felt well.

All of this made sense to a degree, but it placed us in a highly unusual emotional and psychological position. Self-isolating while awaiting a test result was like being suspended in mid-air, floating between wellness and illness. You felt perfectly well but you were being treated as if you were ill. So how, exactly, were you supposed to feel? Well or ill? You might be either or maybe even both.

The first step in dealing with this unfamiliar situation was to recognise that presumptive self-isolation was primarily aimed at protecting others. As the HSE emphasised from the beginning, we really were all in this together. None of us wished to spread the virus.

The second step was to realise that any medical test will always prompt conflicting emotions at the same time or in quick succession. We both want and fear the test result. What if I am sick? And if the test is negative, what caused my symptoms? Will they simply go away?

The rules of logic apply loosely, if at all, in these highly charged situations. Much of what we feel does not make sense, at least at first glance. Recognising this is important. We like to think that our emotions and inner lives have a certain reason to them, but sometimes we need to acknowledge the existence of a tangle of emotions that we simply cannot figure out. So be it. Our logical brains are feeble things at times. Emotions are strident.

To complicate this even more, most of us harbour secret worries that we do not share with anyone. Perhaps, at some level, we know that these anxieties are illogical or exaggerated, but yet we worry. That is the very essence of anxiety: our logical brain might object but the anxiety persists. Most of us know that if we bring ourselves to share these worries with other people we will feel relieved. So will they.

In the midst of the prolonged pandemic, we all had both public and private worries. And while we might dismiss certain anxieties publicly, we carry unease within us until we seek reassurance from a family member or friend. Our brains are excellent at finding new ways to worry.

Perhaps the most astonishing feature of our protracted situation with Covid-19 was that, despite our familiarity with our own anxieties, we often failed to recognise that everyone else was just like us: full of secret worries. All the anxieties and confusions that I feel, other people feel them too.

So, instead of thinking that we are burdening someone else with our worries, we should know that, deep down, other people share our concerns. They need us just as much as we need them. Other people are just the same as us. They *are* us.

The greatest challenges to reaching out and sharing our worries are psychological hesitations rather than physical barriers. Of course, there may be physical barriers too. People who are ill or self-isolating are often most in need of sharing and support. Making the extra effort to connect, possibly by telephone or video-calling, can shift everyone's energies in a more positive direction and away from endless worry.

JULY 2021

July is named after Julius Caesar, the Roman general and statesman. July is a splendid month in many ways. It is the middle of summer. Children are on their school holidays. In the US, it is National Hot Dog Month and National Ice Cream

*Month. What more could anyone want? In the midst of a
pandemic, the July sunshine is especially needed for Ireland's
'outdoor summer'—an unlikely term that recently entered
our vocabulary (and not only ironically). It is not so much the
word 'outdoor' that raises eyebrows as the notion that we have
a 'summer'. Still, on we go.*

The problem with coffee is that I can only have so much of
it. If I have two double espressos within an hour, I become
dizzy and light-headed. Spread evenly over the course of
a morning, however, I consume the entire contents of my
stove-top coffee-pot without difficulty. Pacing is everything.

If I am out and about in a café, I usually sit for quite
a while between coffees, working on my laptop. There is
a soothing pattern to the enterprise: the occasional shot
of caffeine jolts my thinking, quickens my pulse, fires my
typing.

The pandemic sees me sitting outside rather than
inside cafes, but this turns out to be more possible than I
imagined. Maybe the Irish weather is not so bad after all?
Today, there is a gentle July mist as I read Wilde's account
of his Mediterranean voyage.

The *Crusader* left Tenerife on 14 November 1837, visited
Madeira briefly and then headed to Gibraltar. Despite occasional seasickness, conditions on board were quite civilised:

> We dine at three; enjoy our cigar on deck; watch the glories
> of the sunset; speculate on the morrow's weather, and sup
> at seven, after which books, chess and conversation end the

day. But not *every* day. Saturday comes; sweethearts and wives; old Scottish Jem, the boatswain, tunes his fiddle, and the doctor (ship's cook) produces his tambourine; the men dance on deck, and the forecastle sounds with many a song of 'Nelson and Benbow' […] toasts go round, and many a 'Black-eyed Susan' […] is remembered in our 'march upon the mountain-wave'.[12]

Wilde had little time for Gibraltar and left as promptly as he could.[13] The *Crusader* soon anchored in Algiers, to the sounds of 'drums and bugles'.[14] Immediately, however, Wilde and his companions encountered an obstacle that is only too familiar in the era of Covid-19:

> Here [in Algiers] we had to endure that abomination of travelling, a five days' quarantine; as, although there was no sickness at our last port, the great intercourse Gibraltar has with other nations, the French say, renders this necessary.[vi]

Thus the *Crusader* found herself 'stuck in limbo alongside the lazaretto' or isolation hospital for people with infectious diseases, such as leprosy or plague. Then, as now, quarantine was unwanted, unpleasant and difficult to cope with. Today, Covid-19 has made everyone familiar with 'mandatory hotel quarantine', 'stay at home orders' and various other restrictions, but these measures are not new, as Wilde demonstrates. Nor is the displeasure that they trigger:

---

vi   Another point against Gibraltar.

this, too, features in his account. In Algiers, the inspection for the group's release from quarantine was, Wilde said, a 'farce':

> As we were sitting at dinner on the 22nd [of December 1837], a message arrived from the health office to say, we should instantly make our appearance at the lazaretto for examination. The medical attendant was very wrathful at having been delayed a few minutes; if ever he had any French politeness, he must have left it at Marseilles.
>
> This farce consisted in parading all the ship's crew at the same time in a railed-in space, like a parcel of wild beasts in a cage. We were then conducted back to the vessel, and told if we remained in good health until morning, we would get *pratique* [permission to enter the port]. Next morning the health officers came on board in order to fumigate the vessel; a purification so stifling, that we were nearly suffocated.[15]

Despite the indignities of quarantine and their chaotic release from it, Algiers was worth the wait:

> This day was the most exciting I had experienced since I left England. Nothing can exceed the variety and incongruity of costume, and the appearance of the people you meet with in the narrow streets of Algiers ...
>
> All the houses project from the first story upward, which, in more social countries, would have afforded the inhabitants on opposite sides of the streets a comfortable

tete-a-tete; but here they are barricadoed with shutters of close-set lattice-work, admitting little of air, and less of light.

In many places there are perfect arches of stone thrown across the streets, opening here and there to admit a gleam of light, but we were often obliged to grope our way in perfect darkness with outstretched arms, and pacing cautiously along we received into our embrace some portly turbaned Turk, had our toes crushed by the splay-foot of an enormous camel, or were almost squeezed to death against the wall by a heavily-laden donkey.

I could not have believed that so many human habitations could be crowded into so small a compass.[16]

Wilde's quarantine before entering Algiers might have been crudely done but it was necessary. Infectious diseases were an enormous problem in the city's 'civil hospital', which was 'small and crowded to excess'. Malaria was especially common:

The principal diseases now are intermittent fevers, caught from the miasma of the plains. It is of all types ... diarrhoeas, anasarca,[vii] subacute dropsies, and enormous enlargement of the spleen are the usual sequents of this disease [malaria], which is the principal epidemic of the country and by which the French have lost great numbers, especially on the out-stations. The treatment consists in

vii   Severe oedema or fluid retention, it seems.

quinine, given in exceedingly large doses, even to twenty grains; and at times this has the effect of completely cutting short the malady.[17]

Wilde's travails with quarantine were not over. Arriving in Sicily, the *Crusader* applied 'for permission to land' but soon encountered problems:

> After some hours' delay, a board of health, composed of the butchers, bakers, and barbers of the town, made their appearance at the lazaretto, and hearing that we had but just arrived from Barbary [the north coast of Africa, including Algiers], appeared particularly horrified at the thought of admitting so much plague and pestilence amongst them, and consequently imposed a quarantine of twenty-one days upon us; at the same time, each member of the board kindly informed us of their trades and occupations, and solicited our patronage during our captivity. We got off some provisions, and remained at anchor, ready to go to sea the moment the wind favoured.[18]

Quarantine and restrictions were common features of travel in the nineteenth century. The 183 years between Wilde's voyage and our Covid-19 pandemic saw these measures wax and wane, and generally decline in much of the world, especially towards the end of the twentieth century. Certain restrictions never went away fully, however, with some countries requiring specific vaccinations (e.g. yellow fever) in order to enter their territory. More elaborate restrictions and even quarantines might become routine features of travel again if new infections continue to emerge, similar to Covid-19.

Infections have always caused huge suffering, even if many rich countries conveniently ignored this fact over recent decades. In Egypt, Wilde saw yet more evidence of the ravages of infections in Alexandria in the 1830s:

> I was not many minutes in Alexandria until I was forcibly struck with the number of blind people I met at every turn; it is really incredible; the greater number had but one eye, but many others were groping their way through the streets in perfect darkness. Squinting is a very common affection among the people of Alexandria, and the greater number of the lower order are what would be termed 'blear-eyed'; and wherever we went we discovered lamentable traces of the ravages of ophthalmia [inflammation of the eye].[19]

These observations triggered Wilde's interest in trachoma, an infectious cause of blindness, and led to his lifelong interest in ophthalmology or disorders of the eye.[20] In many ways, his subsequent career in medicine was largely shaped by what he saw on this trip and, especially, the devastation wrought by infections. Almost two decades after the voyage, he explored Ireland's epidemics and pandemics in detail in the 1856 census report. Infections were everywhere.

As a doctor, it is interesting for me to reflect on the factors that lead towards a particular specialty within medicine, be it ophthalmology (Wilde); otorhinolaryngology or ear, nose and throat surgery (also Wilde); general practice (many of my classmates from medical school); psychiatry (me); or any of the myriad other possibilities. In secondary school I wanted to be either an economist or a doctor and, if a doctor, a psychiatrist. I chose the latter but still hanker for the former. I wonder is it too late?[viii]

With international travel out of the question, I—like many people—had to find new ways of occupying my imagination during the Covid-19 pandemic. Thinking about my career choice within medicine was one thing, especially as I saw medical colleagues do amazing work in our intensive care units, emergency departments, general practices, vaccination centres and other locations. Work was also busy in psychiatry, with longer days and fluctuating staff levels owing to self-isolation and other complications of the pandemic. No doubt the current generation of medical students will find their career choices shaped by their experiences during Covid-19, just as Wilde's choices were shaped by his travels in 1837 and 1838.

When Wilde and his colleagues were aboard the *Crusader*, they found diversion and refuge in music. 'Black-eyed Susan', which Wilde mentions by name, is a sea song by English poet John Gay (1685–1732). It recounts Susan's search for her William:

All in the Downs the fleet lay moored,
The streamers waving in the wind,

viii   Yes, it is. Don't even think about it.

When black-eyed Susan came on board;
'Oh, where shall I my true-love find?
Tell me, you jovial sailors, tell me true
If my sweet William sails among your crew.'

William is aboard but must, alas, leave Susan behind. On the plus side, he vows to 'forever true remain':

The boatswain gave the dreadful word,
The sails their swelling bosom spread.
No longer must she stay on board,
They kissed, she sighed, he hung his head.
Her less'ning boat unwilling rows to land:
'Adieu', she cries and waves her lily hand.

Almost three centuries after Gay's death,[ix] nearly two centuries after Wilde's voyage and in the midst of the Covid-19 pandemic, different songs provide consolation. Today's tunes are no less stirring than Gay's ballad.

In 2020, Dua Lipa's *Future Nostalgia* had millions dancing around (and on) their kitchen tables during deepest lockdown. For me, Phoebe Bridgers's *Punisher* and Lana Del Ray's *Chemtrails Over the Country Club* arrived straight from heaven. Old favourites returned to my playlist: Sia, Lorde, random Buddhist chants, Sufi compilations, Indian

---

ix   Gay's tomb displays his own words: 'Life is a jest, and all things show
      it, I thought so once, but now I know it'.

taxi music and, of course, the glorious, critically underappreciated songs of Rita Ora.[x]

This month, July 2021, brings more hope. Certain restrictions ease for people who are vaccinated or recovered from Covid-19. Surely this third wave, which began in December 2020, will be one of the last, thanks to vaccination and the passage of time? The relaxation of public health measures over the summer bodes well, but I will be one of the 'hesitant', not least because of the suffering I have seen—and continue to see—at the hospital. It is clear that, whatever progress we have made, this pandemic is not over yet.

Other coping mechanisms? Much has been said about days and nights spent watching Netflix during Covid-19. Although I love movies, I struggle with TV series. I never got past a few episodes of *The Wire* or *Breaking Bad*.[xi]

During lockdown I had a breakthrough: I watched the first and only season of *Gypsy*, a 2017 series in which Naomi Watts plays a psychotherapist. Watts's patient group bears essentially no relationship to real life, but the series still has a lot going for it: desire, betrayal, chic New York apartments and stunning interiors. It was an oddly compelling form of escapism, as well as being completely ludicrous. Ludicrous is not a problem for me: I watched the complete box-set of James Bond movies during Ireland's first lockdown, so my tolerance for absurdity is high.

---

[x]   Rita Ora's 2018 album *Phoenix* is the most perfect pop record of the decade: fizzy, frothy and unburdened by meaning. A masterpiece.

[xi] Sorry.

Other ways of coping? Mischief Theatre's on-line *Movie Night In* was an enormous help, as the Mischief troupe improvised their way through some impressively silly scenarios suggested by viewers. Like all the best theatre, they made an impossibly skilled task look bewilderingly easy. At one level, coping with restrictions called for the absurd, the trivial and the escapist. With so much worrying news flowing into our lives, switching off was sometimes best achieved by tuning into something absorbing, frivolous and unrelated to Covid-19. Mischief Theatre ticked all the (ridiculous) boxes.[xii]

Around me, I saw my friends and colleagues do likewise: combining pragmatic coping strategies with more and more escapism as the pandemic progressed. Many took to running, cycling and swimming with new-found gusto, but they also watched more TV, looked at different movies and read a wider variety of books. We need both forms of coping in order to get by: day-to-day physical activities and an outlet for our imaginations. If I cannot drink over-priced coffee in New York, at least I can watch Naomi Watts do so in *Gypsy*. If I cannot travel to the theatre, at least I can watch *Mischief Movie Night In* on-line.

Some of our coping mechanisms are rational, others are not. This is no surprise. Covid-19 and our anxieties about it present an enormous challenge to the usual mix of logic and emotion that governs our behaviour. In the midst of a world turned upside down, logic is not the only way forward, nor even necessarily the best one.[21]

xii   Thank you, Mischief.

Aristotle reportedly said that a human being is a 'rational animal'. If he truly said this, then he was both right and wrong. He was right to the extent that humans have enormously complex brains, comprising over 86 billion nerve cells along with many more supporting structures, brain chemicals and various other cells. And, for the most part, we use our brains to good effect: understanding the world, solving problems and communicating with each other in astonishingly subtle ways. Our brains are extraordinary.

But Aristotle was wrong if he thought that human beings are entirely rational. There is growing evidence that many of the decisions that we believe to be logical and rational are deeply influenced by emotion and irrational beliefs.

There is nothing wrong with emotions shaping what we do, but it is useful to recognise when this is happening. The first step is for us to become more aware of our feelings as they occur. Clearly labelling each emotion in our heads helps us to recognise how we feel and how strong our emotions really are. This became very important during the pandemic, as emotions changed rapidly, especially in the opening months of 2020.

Second, we should work hard to accept our emotions, regardless of what they are. We cannot negotiate directly with feelings, so we need to accept our anger, our frustration, our fear and our happiness. We should, however, remain confident that we can handle any emotion that arises: these are all transient feelings and they will pass.

Third, it is useful to try to figure out why we feel this way *right now*. Is there a trigger? Sometimes there is and sometimes there is not. It is especially useful to identify when negative emotions have no clear trigger or focus. This helps them to dissipate.

The Covid-19 outbreak triggered strong emotions in many people. These were commonly centred on anxiety, anger, fear and sadness. It is important to recognise these feelings, even as they persist today, long after the pandemic began.

It is also useful to recognise that Covid-19 placed many people in unfamiliar situations which provoke unusual emotions. For example, many countries asked people with symptoms to 'self-isolate'. In some countries 'limited social interaction' was advised, while general 'social distancing' came into effect elsewhere.

While all of these steps are effective public health measures, they create unusual social and emotional situations with which most people are unfamiliar. Quarantine has similar effects, often resulting in fear of infection, frustration, boredom and annoyance at lack of information. There can be problems with stigma, finances and tensions in relationships, as well as anger towards people from epicentres of the outbreak and towards governments for perceived inaction.

These problems can be mitigated by terminating public health measures when they are no longer necessary, providing adequate information and supplies to those affected, improving communication (using technology where possible) and, for children, continuing schooling and education as best as is feasible. Emotional awareness is vital. These are unusual circumstances at a time of unique emotional intensity. Labelling our emotions and checking in on how we feel can help greatly as we navigate these challenges.

It is useful to remember that emotions can disguise themselves as behaviours or facts—and can therefore mislead us. Often, emotions manifest as behaviours that we poorly understand (even in ourselves), as 'facts' that upset us (and likely are not true), or as a general sense of confusion about what is going on and how we feel about it.[22]

The key to dealing with these distressing situations is to recognise that we can have several conflicting emotions at the same time or in quick succession. It is helpful to practise simply sitting with uncomfortable emotional states—tolerating distress without trying to understand it fully. An activity like meditation helps greatly. Meditation is often described as a 'practice'. This is true. Even meditation masters, after decades of contemplation, still 'practise'. Imperfection is part of the deal.

As well as reflecting on your own emotions, it is helpful to talk to other people about how you are feeling. It is equally helpful to listen to others who are experiencing the same emotions as you but might express them differently. Take time to let them explain. Once we listen deeply, we see how similar we all are. This is especially important at times of threat, illness or personal loss, such as now. Direct, truthful communication is vital, once we are just as willing to listen as we are to speak. In other words, if you want to be heard, listen.

Finally, it is always good to escape, if only in our minds. When we had to stay within 5km of our homes, I took to reading old books about travels around Ireland, describing places that lay just beyond my tightening horizon. Living in Dublin but born in Galway, and very taken by Wilde's book about Connemara,[23] I was similarly struck by Harold Speakman's account of the west in his 1926 memoir *Here's Ireland*:

> Northwest from Galway town lies Connemara. It is a land of red skirts and a thousand wrinkled faces. It is a land where girls don't forget to smile at you any more than they do in Kerry, and where horses, carrying huge loads of whatever they have to carry on their two-wheeled carts, work for their masters up and down the hills with great good will. It is a land where those hills are such an intense cobalt blue, and the sky is such an intense cerulean blue, and the clouds are so white and the wind-pressed foliage of oak and elm and juniper is so black against the hillsides that the whole thing becomes a sort of pain.[24]

Wilde, too, appreciated Connemara, but his travels in 1837 and 1838 were a little more exotic. After Alexandria, he explored much of the rest of Egypt: the tombs, the pyramids and the city of Cairo. There was plenty of history, archaeology and medicine to feed his hunger for knowledge. He saw a 'revolting and disgusting' 'mad-house' in Cairo,[25] as well as an unusual consequence of the bubonic plague that ravaged Egypt from 1834 to 1836, shortly before he arrived there:

> A dog at the hotel attracted our notice; it had a peculiar description of palsy, an interrupted and sudden seizure of

the body, as if it had received an electric shock; the limbs bending under it, and the whole body trembling violently for a second, when it again appeared in perfect health. About six months previous, a Frank had the plague, and none would go near him; this dog, however, never left him, and carried to him whatever was left for his use; and was also in the constant practice of licking the plague sores. The man recovered, but the dog fell ill; boils, analogous to those of the plague, broke out on it; it remained in the apartment of the man it had so lately nursed, and finally, it, too, escaped; but it recovered with the affection I describe. It has since taken up its quarters at the Hotel de Jardin, and has become, by its history, a general favourite. In other respects, it is in good health.[26]

Everywhere that Wilde looked, he saw plague, illness and the consequences of infection. It is no surprise that he later focused so sharply on these themes in his 1856 census report. It is even less surprising that his work speaks so eloquently to us today, in the era of Covid-19. Infection is eternal.

AUGUST 2021

August is named after Augustus Caesar, the first Roman emperor, who reigned from 27 BC until he died in AD 14. In the US, August is National Immunisation Awareness Month, which is especially appropriate this year, in the midst of the Covid-19 pandemic. August is also National Goat Cheese Month and

Sandwich Month, so there's a lot here for me. Even better, this month brings the end of summer. I like when autumn appears on the horizon. Ralph Waldo Emerson is of a similar mind: 'When summer opens, I see how fast it matures and fear it will be short; but after the heats of July and August, I am reconciled, like one who has had his swing, to the cool of autumn'. Me too. It's time.

August brings my birthday. This year moves me ever closer to the end of my fifth decade and prompts some reflection. Birthdays usually float past without triggering any particular thoughts, but perhaps the uncertainties of Covid-19 change the context this year. It is not that the passage of time troubles me (that would be pointless), but the losses associated with the pandemic contribute to a certain reflectiveness. This August just feels different.

More specifically, it occurs to me that my forties and thirties have been busy with all kinds of things, but I am not entirely certain how I spent my twenties, from a professional perspective. Not really. My curriculum vitae tells me I was a medical student and worked in a seamless series of jobs as a junior hospital doctor (all of which is true), but I remember little about the thoughts I had about work or what I imagined I was doing with my career. Sometimes I wish I could say that my twenties were lost in a haze of hedonistic excess, but I most certainly cannot.[xiii]

---

xiii Should anyone ever see three movies in one day at the Irish Film Institute? I have, and will probably do so again. That does not mean it is right, obviously.

I might have had too much coffee over those busy years, but let's be charitable and put that down to anthropological exploration rather than addiction. Wilde pointed to the insights available in coffee outlets in 1838: 'How much of life and manners are to be seen in a coffee-shop!', he observed.[27] I could not agree more.

Wilde wrote these words in Cairo, in the midst of his Mediterranean adventures, while enjoying the delights of an Egyptian coffee-house:

> The solemn visages and portly persons of the turbaned visitors are revealed in momentary glimpses, as the veil of smoke clears away, upon the renewal of a pipe or the sipping of a cup of coffee; and the Arab story-teller, singing his tale from the beauties of the thousand-and-one nights, or some popular romance, in all the glowing imagery, all the rapid enunciation, and all the touching pathos of an eastern bard. 'Tis true, that as I sat and listened among the crowd I could not understand one word he uttered; but I saw the fire of his eye, I felt the power though not the meaning of his language, and caught the spirit of his song, though I could not fully appreciate the letter; for such is eloquence—proudest, noblest of the innate powers of man, which all can feel.

After Egypt, Wilde travelled to Asia Minor, Syria, Palestine, Jerusalem and Greece. Everywhere he went, he saw more history, more archaeology and more evidence of the impact of infections on different countries and civilisations. On the

Greek island of Rhodes, the effects of leprosy and plague were immediately apparent:

> Here I first witnessed the true eastern leprosy: for several unfortunate creatures afflicted with this terrific malady are congregated on the island, and are to be met sitting by the wayside begging. A Greek chief, many years ago, with a feeling and humanity that does honour to the name of Greece, even in her most degenerate state, purchased a small tract of land in the interior of the island, for the purpose of affording lepers a secluded and a comfortable asylum, and thither they come from all the neighbouring places […]
>
> Owing to a want of cleanliness—a quarantine and due precaution—and its intercourse with the Porte, plague was formerly a constant visitor here; and in the last attack it is said to have taken off nearly a third of the Turkish population, while the Greeks suffered comparatively little.[28]

Everywhere that Wilde went: illness, infection, plague. The evidence was endless. Infection was ubiquitous. How could we forget this now? How could Covid-19 take us totally by surprise?

Eventually, Wilde and his fellow travellers made their way home, arriving in Kingstown (Dún Laoghaire) more than eight months after the start of their epic voyage:

> On the morning of the 3rd of June [1838], we entered Kingstown harbour. The hour was early; the inhabitants had not yet stirred. There was scarcely a vessel in port.

A thick mist hung over Killiney hill, and everything looked lonely and deserted; but still it was with a beating heart I hailed that shore, to me,

'More dear in its storms, its clouds, and its showers,
Than the rest of this world in its sunniest hours.'[29]

Like many travellers, Wilde was happy to have journeyed and happy to be home. He was fortunate not to acquire any of the infectious diseases that he encountered along the way and to return to Ireland in good health. Not all travellers are so lucky.

Wilde's career in medicine was shaped by his trip and, especially, by the impact of plagues, pandemics and the lack of medical care that he saw in so many countries. These experiences left a lasting impression in his memory and on his mind. Like many doctors, his motivation in his profession was a complex mix of compassion, scientific enquiry and excitement at the possibility of helping others. For Wilde, knowledge was a necessary requirement for care, and care was, of course, the very purpose of medicine.

Today, in early August 2021, as the Covid-19 pandemic subsides in certain rich countries, many of the issues identified by Wilde on his 1837 trip remain apparent. Infectious diseases still incur enormous cost, as rich countries recently rediscovered and poor countries never forgot. Pandemics continue to transform societies, often in unpredictable ways. Lack of basic medical care still ends millions of lives prematurely, and never more so than during a pandemic. In Ireland, we are more fortunate than some of the countries that Wilde visited, owing to the rapid implementation of public health measures at the start of Covid-19, and the arrival of vaccines that are effective and safe and can be scaled up. Again, not everyone is so lucky, even today.

Following his return in 1838, Wilde threw himself into work with gusto, building on both his medical qualifications and his burgeoning interest in infections. He took rooms at 199 Great Brunswick Street in Dublin and began to write his two-volume account of his travels, along with other learned papers.[30] Wilde was busy: working constantly, writing furiously and reading essays at the Royal Irish Academy, the Royal Dublin Society and the British Association. His book of travels appeared in 1840. I am fascinated by it, even now, over a century and a half later. Despite some regrettable passages that inevitably reveal the prejudices of the times, most of his text is literate, logical and involving.

Today Great Brunswick Street, where Wilde had his rooms, is known as Pearse Street. It is a remarkably busy thoroughfare along the side of Trinity College, Dublin, where I work. Further up Pearse Street from the main campus, the Trinity Biomedical Sciences Institute (TBSI) houses Trinity's Centres for Cancer Drug Discovery, Medical Device Technologies and Translational Medicine, along with various other research activities. TBSI also delivers the early years of the university's undergraduate medical course. This is where students get the scientific and pre-clinical knowledge they need before moving on to their clinical education in teaching hospitals and GP surgeries linked with the medical school.

Sitting in the Science Gallery on Pearse Street today, intoxicated by one espresso too many, I am struck by the changes that have taken place since Wilde had rooms here in 1838. The street is transformed beyond recognition: it is busier, brasher and considerably more frenetic than in Wilde's time. Medicine, too, has changed immeasurably, and research technology has advanced at pace. What would Wilde make of these developments?

Foolishly draining yet another espresso, I conclude that Wilde would be dismayed by the aggressive traffic, astonished but not surprised at advances in medicine and taken aback by the technology in research centres such as TBSI. He would likely collapse with disbelief were he to understand the research capabilities of even a single laboratory in the building.[xiv]

Even so, I am confident that Wilde would recognise the spirit of care and enquiry that lies at the heart of medical practice and research today. He would be instantly familiar with the impact of illness that drives research, continued efforts to explain the biological mechanisms of disease and the sustained desire to improve our understandings of the determinants, distribution and treatment of infections around the world, including Covid-19. Technology might evolve but some things never change. Wilde would understand this.

xiv   Seriously, it is one impressive place.

Wilde would also recognise the strengths and weaknesses of public health measures for controlling infectious diseases, such as distancing, isolation and quarantine. Pandemic responses still depend on these steps today. These measures might date from medieval times but they remain stubbornly effective. The Covid-19 pandemic has proven definitively that these blunt interventions still play a role in managing outbreaks, preventing greater spread of infection and saving lives. Combined with vaccination, these interventions have made an enormous difference.

As if to prove this point, Taoiseach Micheál Martin makes a speech on the last day of August 2021, announcing substantial easing of restrictions over the coming months as a result of these measures:

The journey through the Covid pandemic up to this point has been one like no other. We've had to accept restrictions on our personal freedoms that would have been unthinkable just a couple of years ago. Never before have we confronted a public health and economic challenge of this scale, and which has continued to rapidly evolve.

The Government has directly intervened in the economy and provided massive direct supports in a manner and on a scale that is simply unprecedented. All of this, and much more, was necessary because our number one priority had to be the protection of people's lives and public health.

We were also determined to do whatever we had to do, to keep as much of our society and economy intact until we could safely emerge from restrictions. But protecting lives and public health has demanded policies which have often been frustrating.[31]

Martin acknowledges that Ireland has 'pushed forward with one of the most determined and comprehensive vaccination programmes in the world', made possible by 'extraordinary scientific effort on a global scale'. This 'changes the dynamic utterly', he says. As a result, Ireland can continue to open up. He duly outlines a series of measures that will see a degree of normality return to Irish life. Could the dark times be coming to an end? Hope is both dangerous and necessary. While we sometimes worry that hope can lead to disappointment, it is essential if we are to move forward, especially now. We have no choice but to hope. And so we do.

American writer Lawrence Wright explores these themes in his superb book *The Plague Year: America in the Time of Covid*.[32] As he tells the story of Covid-19 in the US, he examines the US government's response to the pandemic, the arrival of vaccines and the hope they inspire. Like me, Wright scarcely felt the jab himself. It was a quiet miracle.

Nevertheless, as Wright shows, initial enthusiasm is often followed by new anxieties. No sooner were vaccines being rolled out than more variants of the virus emerged. The seemingly endless story of Covid-19 took new turns. Would it ever end? Would hope be justified? Optimism sustained?

Despite the new complexities documented so carefully by Wright, vaccines continued to perform strongly, and still do so today. Public health systems continue to respond to the evolving threat of the virus. Sadly, there are further deaths and new cases, but progress is undeniable: in countries where vaccines are available, the pandemic is in decline.

Coming out of a time like this is difficult for many people. Survival is a cause for celebration, but survival brings its own complexities. Martin acknowledges this in his speech at the end of August. Many people experience complicated emotions as life restarts without their loved ones who have died:

> As we move into this new phase, it will be a time of trepidation for some as they re-engage with activities and resume old habits after a long period of isolation. We will be bringing forward a health and well-being programme to help people reconnect. Others will be nervous as they move to reopen long-closed venues and projects.
>
> It will be a time of anticipation and relief for others as they finally get back to doing what they do best, particularly in our arts and entertainment sectors. As patrons and event goers, we will be delighted to enjoy them again.
>
> For many others, it will be a time of reflection, and sadness. For while we have come to this point in the pandemic with fewer deaths than many other countries, we have still paid a terrible price.

As Wilde knew, infections always carry a 'terrible price'. He saw this in the bubonic plague and leprosy that shaped the countries he visited in 1837 and 1838, in the epidemics and pandemics that he documented in his census report in 1856, and—most of all—in the meningitis that likely took the life of his beautiful daughter, Isola, in 1867. As Wright points out in his book, the losses of Covid-19, too, need to be acknowledged, if we are to cope with the pandemic and navigate the changed, new world in which we hope to live.

Many politicians finish their Covid-19 speeches with messages of hope. Martin does likewise today:

> Over centuries we have demonstrated that as a nation, we have great resilience and ingenuity. We have weathered many storms, we've borne many ordeals, we've faced down many threats and we have seized many opportunities. Over the last eighteen months, we have drawn on all of that, and we have endured.
>
> Now, we will push on to complete our vaccination programme, including a winter booster programme that will commence in the coming weeks. And we will play our full and active part in making vaccines available to vulnerable people all around the world.
>
> We will rebuild our economy and renew our society. We will do these and all the other things with renewed energy and determination, with personal freedoms restored and our country, we hope, emerging from this most extraordinary period in our history.

Martin's words are well spoken and necessary. It is especially heartening to hear that 'we will play our full and active part in making vaccines available to vulnerable people all around the world'. I hope this is true.

As August 2021 ends, hope is palpable, if fragile. Maybe that is always the way, especially when hope has been dashed so many times before.

Albert Einstein advised us to 'learn from yesterday, live for today, hope for tomorrow. The important thing is not to stop questioning.' Covid-19 raised so many issues that there is little chance that anyone will 'stop questioning'. There will be reviews, analyses and enquiries into government responses all over the world. So be it: it is important to examine every crisis with care and extract lessons for the future. What could we have done better? How might we have saved more lives?

Wilde performed a similar examination in his 1856 census report, and we need to do the same thing now. This is another one of Wilde's lessons: we must face the past, and understand it as well as possible, if we are to shape the future with confidence and knowledge.

It is important to be both hopeful and realistic, and to live in the world as we find it, not as we imagine it to be. US President Woodrow Wilson saw hope as an essential component of both growing within the world we have today and building the kind of world we want to create tomorrow:

You are not here merely to make a living. You are here in order to enable the world to live more amply, with greater vision, with a finer spirit of hope and achievement. You are here to enrich the world, and you impoverish yourself if you forget the errand.

The Covid-19 pandemic resulted in all kinds of impoverishment: lives lost, health impaired, education disrupted, livelihoods ruined, dreams denied, hopes diminished. Nevertheless, despite everything, we are still here to enrich the world. August 2021 brought a new sense of hope. Many people coped with the pandemic better than they might have expected. Despite the battering, we will thrive again.

3. AUTUMN 2021:
NOT COPING

'Difficulties are things that show a person what they are.'

—*Epictetus*

*T*his chapter starts in September 2021, when public *health restrictions are eased and hope grows that the end of the pandemic is in sight—or, at least, imaginable. Vaccines help enormously, reducing risks of infection, transmission, illness and death. Even so, the toll of Covid-19 has grown beyond understanding: millions have died, billions have suffered. Research indicates that one person in every five has significant psychological distress. Among healthcare workers the rate is doubled. These figures are remarkably consistent across countries, including Ireland. But there is also widespread evidence of strength, coping and resilience: after all, four people in every five do* not *report disabling psychological problems, even with the world in flames around us. These themes are explored in this chapter, along with William Wilde's obsessional account of the final illness of Jonathan Swift. The end of November 2021*

sees Covid-19 cases rising again across Europe and the psycho-
logical challenge intensifying once more. The hope that vaccines
brought remains strong, but will this ever actually end?

SEPTEMBER 2021

September, the ninth month, derives its name from the Latin
word septem, *meaning 'seven'. It was originally the seventh*
month in the calendar of Romulus, dating from around 750 BC.
September is a time of return and beginning, the opening of the
academic year in much of the world, and the start of the ecclesi-
astical year for the Eastern Orthodox Church. Philosophers and
poets are filled with praise for and excitement about the season
and the month. For William Wordsworth, 'wild is the music of
autumnal winds amongst the faded woods'. For Albert Camus,
'autumn is a second spring when every leaf is a flower'. For
Voltaire, 'wine is the divine juice of September'. Thoreau finds
hope in nature: 'Happily we bask in this warm September sun,
which illuminates all creatures'.

I am not exactly basking in September sun today, but there
is light. The first of the month brings hope.

Newspapers respond joyously to Taoiseach Micheál
Martin's announcement that Covid-19 restrictions start
to ease today. The *Irish Times* headline reads: 'Taoiseach
sets out timetable to lift remaining Covid restrictions'.
The government plan is set out on the front page: public
transport returns to full capacity today; other restrictions

will ease gradually over coming months. The newspaper's editorial talks about 'preparing for the new normal'. The front page of the *Irish Examiner* quotes Martin: 'The days of hope are here'. Are they? It seems almost too good to be true.

The question in everyone's minds is whether this can last. We have had optimistic days earlier in this pandemic and we have been disappointed. Why is this time special?

The front-page headline of the *Irish Independent* cuts to the core of why it's different this time round: 'Booster shots key to plans for ending all restrictions'. Vaccination has an astonishing impact, with promise of more to come. The vaccines brought hope, virtually overnight. They did not solve all our problems, but they transformed the situation in hospitals and nursing homes, among front-line staff and across the population generally—at least for those who can access vaccines.

The idea of salvation is traditionally a religious one: salvation by the gods, by our own good deeds or as a reward for past virtues. Salvation by science is relatively new—or, rather, it feels new every time it happens. Today, vaccines slot into the salvation role with ease, reducing risks of infection, transmission, illness and death. Even people who are not vaccinated derive benefits from those who are. For some, this is an extension of the miracle. For others, it is involuntary altruism: protecting others by protecting ourselves.

In mid-September, Ben Quinn in *The Guardian* points out just how much of an impact the vaccines make:

People who were fully vaccinated accounted for just 1.2% of all deaths involving Covid-19 in England in the first seven months of [2021]. The figures, published by the Office for National Statistics (ONS), have been seized on as proof of the success of the vaccine programme […] No vaccine is 100% effective against Covid-19, and health authorities have said some deaths of vaccinated individuals are to be expected. Public Health England (PHE) has estimated that two-dose effectiveness against hospital admission with infections from the Delta variant—which is the UK's dominant variant—has been around 94%.[1]

Of the 51,281 Covid-19 deaths in England between 2 January and 2 July 2021, just 640 were of people who had received two vaccination doses. This is astonishing. Vaccines work better than anyone might have expected. In fact, their effectiveness is so great that we can almost lose sight of some of the most troubling aspects of the pandemic that still persist, despite our new-found hope. Today, as we head into our second winter with the virus, these problems are worth remembering.

First, even with the benefits of vaccination kicking in, the cumulative losses to date are almost beyond understanding. Take a rich, developed country like the United States. This month brings news that more Americans have died of Covid-19 than died in the 1918 'flu pandemic.[2] The US makes up 5 per cent of the world's population but accounts for 14 per cent of the world's 4.7 million deaths from Covid-19 to date. So, while vaccines are hugely effective, they come too late for many, not everyone gets access, and they are not equally or fairly distributed around the world.[3]

In the past, I often wondered what it would be like to live through a global emergency or worldwide catastrophe, such as a world war, the 1918 'flu pandemic or one of the epidemics, tragedies or cosmic events outlined by Wilde in his colourful account of Ireland's history. Now I know. The Covid-19 pandemic is as dramatic an event as any generation has experienced and I have lived through it from the start.

The most startling aspect for me is how distant the pandemic sometimes feels, even though I work in a hospital. Some days it can seem surreal, if only for a few moments. Then, abruptly, the enormity of the outbreak comes back into focus, when I hear that a family member or friend is affected, a patient develops Covid-19 or I read an especially powerful media report. It intrigues me that I can focus on the day-to-day challenges presented at work and put the terrifying global picture to the back of my mind for periods of time, so that the enormity of the pandemic feels oddly distant at times. Millions have died, but my chief concern most mornings is remembering to bring a face-covering to wear as I cross the carpark into work.

Surely this is just plain wrong? Should I not be continually gripped, heart and soul, by the global emergency? Utterly paralysed by the tragedy unfolding around me? I am not. For much of the time, I focus on detail: where did I put my box of face-masks, have I washed my hands and do I have clean scrubs ready for work tomorrow? The global picture is too big for me to carry in my head every moment of every day.

The other time that the pandemic comes into sharp focus for me is when I am asked about its impact on mental health. Given that I work as a psychiatrist, this is a question I get asked a lot by patients, families, friends and journalists.

Journalists mostly start by asking whether the psychological impact of the pandemic and public restrictions has been ignored. I think they want me to say 'Yes', but the truth is that the impact of Covid-19 on mental health is never far from the headlines. Perhaps I focus selectively on this theme when I hear it in the media, and maybe other people ignore it, but it seems to me that politicians and commentators speak frequently about the psychological effects of the pandemic and public health restrictions. My own clinical work confirms Wilde's view that infections always carry a heavy price, both physically and mentally. Even our politicians realise this now, it seems to me.

But is this just empty rhetoric from our leaders? Politicians often invoke 'mental health' when they struggle for other things to say, hoping that simply uttering the words 'mental health' will earn them admiration and respect. They are rarely held to account for precisely what they mean when they say that 'mental health' is important. What do they propose doing? What actions will they take, and when?

On top of these usual questions, the pandemic prompted a new set of queries about psychological well-being. Exactly how have Covid-19 and our pandemic responses affected mental health? Who is most at risk? Where is the evidence for this? What should we do?

From the earliest stages of the pandemic, health professionals and researchers studied the psychological and psychiatric impact of the unfolding catastrophe with great care.[4] It was clearly going to have an impact. By September 2021, over a year and a half into the pandemic, the results of these studies were remarkably consistent: the pandemic affected mental health very broadly right around the world.[5] The evidence for this is vast, so let's break it down and start with the pandemic's impact on the general population, before considering special groups such as healthcare workers. And, like the pandemic, let's start in China.

The first case of Covid-19 was identified in Wuhan in late December 2019. As the infection spread, one on-line study of 1,210 people across 194 Chinese cities in January and February 2020 found that 54 per cent of people rated the psychological impact of the outbreak as moderate or severe, 29 per cent reported moderate to severe anxiety symptoms, and 17 per cent reported moderate to severe depressive symptoms.[6] These findings were not unexpected: the panic and uncertainty associated with an outbreak such as Covid-19 inevitably make us anxious and concerned about the future. Most people had never experienced anything like this before. Nobody knew what might happen next. Many feared the worst. Already, some were bereaved.

As these research results filtered out from China in early 2020, the big surprise for me was not that so many people

were struggling emotionally but that significant numbers did *not* report anxiety or depression. Almost half the
people surveyed said that they were coping well, without
significant psychological problems. How could this be?
Did they not see what was unfolding around them? The
world was in flames, with no sign of relief, and they were
keeping calm and carrying on? Many were distressed, but
many were not.

It seemed extraordinary to me, but the results from
China were confirmed by an on-line survey of 21,207
people in Spain, conducted a week after lockdown began
there, in March 2020. The Spanish results were similar to
those from China: four people in every ten had depressive
responses to recent events, four in ten had avoidant behaviour, and three in ten reported stress.[7] Again, I was surprised
that the figures were not higher: this was a time of unique
anxiety and unprecedented stress. While many people were
struggling and needed support, well over half of the population in Spain and elsewhere appeared to be coping without
significant anxiety, stress or depressive symptoms. This was
impressive.

What about Ireland? Between March and June 2020
(during restrictions) one on-line study of 847 members
of the Irish public reported significant increases in symptoms of depression, anxiety and stress.[8] Again, this was
to be expected: nobody had experienced anything like
this before. Another study, performed by researchers at
Maynooth University and Trinity College, surveyed 1,000
people in March and April 2020 (also during restrictions)

and found that 41 per cent reported feeling lonely, 23 per cent reported clinically meaningful depression, 20 per cent reported anxiety and 18 per cent had symptoms of post-traumatic stress.[9]

These findings do not mean that one fifth of the population was mentally ill. Most people cope with difficulty by reaching out to family and friends, exercising more, changing their lifestyles and doing things they have always done in times of stress or trouble. We are resourceful people, especially when we support each other.[10]

This is not mental illness. This is a normal response to an abnormal situation. It can be highly distressing but, with personal assistance and support, most people get through it. Over-medicalising this kind of distress disempowers people who would otherwise cope quite well. It also de-emphasises social and political solutions to much of this suffering: strengthening communities, protecting employment, supporting businesses, providing financial assistance to those who need it and implementing public health measures that earn the public's trust.

So, while the numbers were high—between a quarter and a third of the Irish population reported psychological problems—the rates were not nearly as high as might have been expected. Many people were coping with the challenge. Distress was widespread but, for most people, not disabling. A majority of people set the global picture aside for much of the time and carried on as best they could.

Despite the clear logic of this approach and the lack of any practical alternative, I was still surprised that more people were not severely anxious or depressed. It was remarkable.

If, prior to Covid-19, someone had told me that there would be a global pandemic, millions would die, societies would lock down, economies would grind to a virtual halt, schools would close and international travel would cease, I would have imagined that nobody could cope with such a situation. I would have been wrong. Our resilience and coping mechanisms proved stronger than I thought. Many people had psychological problems, but an equal number—or more—did not. We are stronger than we think. We were always stronger, but we never realised it until now.

In addition, a great many people reached out for help during those opening months of the pandemic, connecting with family, friends, colleagues and healthcare profession-als. A survey of 195 psychiatrists conducted by the College of Psychiatrists of Ireland in May and June 2020 found that a majority of psychiatrists reported increased referrals for generalised anxiety (79 per cent of psychiatrists reported an increase), health anxiety (72 per cent), depression (57 per cent) and panic (54 per cent) compared to earlier in the pandemic.[11] The College commented:

> Strikingly, when compared with numbers *prior to the lock-down*, 1 in 3 consultant psychiatrists [35%] saw an increase in the number of emergency referrals and 50% cited the number of patients experiencing a relapse of mental illness as having increased […] This mental health curve arising needs to be urgently addressed and flattened by the incom-

ing government with a national multi-sectorial taskforce, clear leadership and doubling of the funding to mental health services required.[12]

Over the course of the pandemic, there was a particular increase in need for child and adolescent mental health services (CAMHS), placing that service under considerable pressure.[13] There were reports of increased attendances at primary care counselling services, and increased presentations to emergency departments and specialist mental health services, especially with eating disorders. Following an immediate reduction after lockdown, there was a sustained increase in emergency department presentations by children for acute mental health care and referrals to CAMHS.

For both children and adults, the reasons for these presentations included anxiety about Covid-19 itself and the effects of restrictions, such as quarantine, which can contribute to confusion, anger and post-traumatic stress symptoms.[14] Particular stressors include longer duration of quarantine or isolation, infection fears, boredom, frustration, inadequate supplies or information, financial loss and stigma. All of these concerns were in clear evidence from the start of the pandemic, especially following the implementation of public health restrictions that were necessary for all but challenging for many.

The initial impact of the public health measures was a decrease in presentations to mental health services rather than an increase, because many people stayed at home despite their psychological and psychiatric problems. Provisional figures showed that hospital presentations for self-harm fell by 25 per cent in April 2020 (shortly after the pandemic began) compared to April 2019.[15] This, however, was in the context of a 40 per cent fall in *all* presentations to hospitals for any reason over this time. In those early months, most people were too scared to go anywhere. Only the very sick went to hospital, and this applied to people with concerns about their mental health as well as those with physical symptoms.

In June 2020 the College of Psychiatrists of Ireland noted that, despite the initial decline in referrals for mental health problems, workloads soon started to build, and it became increasingly difficult to deliver effective care in the context of the pandemic:

> Although referrals were down in the initial phase of the virus, psychiatrists have seen an increased workload for the duration of the pandemic thus far, with teams continually adapting services to incorporate new technologies and delivery of assessment via telephone/video-link, adjusted referral pathways and colleagues being on leave.
>
> Many [consultant psychiatrists] commented that while consultant staff and multi-disciplinary team members had adapted rapidly to changes and new referral pathways, these adaptations have left clear staffing deficits exposed.
>
> Along with precautions around the spread of Covid-19 in healthcare settings has come the widescale rollout of patient assessment using telepsychiatry methods. However,

67 per cent of 87 respondents who answered the IT [information technology] questions [in the College survey] felt they were ill equipped to conduct some/most or all duties from an IT perspective. Respondents noted no availability or poor signal of WiFi in offices, and that personal home WiFi connections were also causing issues with the use of telepsychiatry assessment.[16]

I was one of those psychiatrists, relying on home WiFi for meetings and teaching commitments, although, like my colleagues, I continued to attend the hospital for patient consultations, ward rounds and clinical work. This combination of home working and going to the hospital was complicated and filled with questions. Is this trip to work really necessary? How can I minimise risk? What if I bring Covid-19 home? The issues were endless and were shared by many people, not just healthcare workers, over the course of the pandemic.

In parallel with these daily personal struggles, the broader picture about how we were coping with world events became clearer. Any number of research studies confirmed those early results from China and Spain: the combined effect of the Covid-19 pandemic and associated restrictions was that approximately one person in every five in the general population had significantly increased psychological distress, mostly symptoms of anxiety and depression. Not everyone was affected equally: particular risk factors included being female and living alone.[17] In addition, another high-risk group for mental ill health rapidly emerged and should not, in retrospect, have been a surprise: people infected with Covid-19.

Experience with severe acute respiratory syndrome (SARS) suggested that an infection such as SARS or Covid-19 could affect both physical and mental health, sometimes severely and sometimes in a lasting way. Among patients hospitalised with SARS in Hong Kong in 2003, 59 per cent fulfilled criteria for a mental illness thirty months later, mostly post-traumatic stress disorder or depression.[18] This was a large proportion of those who contracted SARS and suggested clear cause for concern with Covid-19.

Similar evidence soon emerged of increased levels of depression, anxiety and post-traumatic stress among people who tested positive for Covid-19.[19] One Chinese study of 103 Covid-19 patients hospitalised with mild symptoms of the infection found that 60 per cent reported depression and 55 per cent reported anxiety, compared to 31 per cent and 22 per cent (respectively) of people without Covid-19.[20] The level of inflammation caused by the virus was correlated with the level of depression in Covid-19 patients, linking the infection with their psychological distress.

A large US study of medical records found that the incidence of any psychiatric diagnosis fourteen to ninety days after a Covid-19 diagnosis was over 18 per cent—almost one in five.[21] From a mental health perspective, this was SARS all over again. It seemed that a second wave of psychological problems linked to Covid-19 would soon emerge, as was seen in the aftermath of previous epidemics and pandemics, so carefully documented by Wilde.

With Covid-19, there are two links between infection and mental ill health. First, the virus itself can have a significant effect on the brain.[22] Most infections, such as influenza, increase the risk of anxiety and depression following an episode of physical illness. Covid-19 can clearly do likewise, and this biological effect contributes to the risk of mental illness during the months after infection, even following complete physical recovery. This continues to be the case today: Covid-19 has a sustained neuro-biological effect in some people, contributing to mental ill health. Most are fine, but some are not.

Second, and probably equally important, is the psychological trauma of being diagnosed and hospitalised with Covid-19, especially at the start of the pandemic. Illness is always challenging, and hospitalisation can be more so, but the uncertainties of the early months of this pandemic were on a different level to anything previously experienced by this generation in many (but not all) parts of the world. Nobody knew what the outcomes of Covid-19 were, how it was best treated or how to manage the risk of people with the virus infecting other patients, their families or healthcare workers. Hospitalisation at this stage was deeply traumatic for many, and likely linked to the risk of psychological problems later on.

Against this background, it was clear that the best way to limit the negative mental health effects of Covid-19 was by preventing infection in the first place, through a combination of personal responsibility (insofar as possible), public health measures (implemented by governments) and vaccines (when they came on stream). Distress associated with restrictions could be diminished by maintaining restrictions for no longer than required, providing clear rationales and information about protocols, ensuring sufficient supplies and reminding the public about the benefits of these public health measures.[23]

For those infected and hospitalised, liaison psychiatry services were vital for providing mental health care while in hospital, as well as multi-disciplinary follow-up after discharge. There was also a demonstrated need for primary care (GP) and secondary mental health services for people with longer-term psychiatric problems as a result of Covid-19, including children, adolescents, adults, older people, people with intellectual disabilities and various other groups.[24] Clearly, many needed help.

Although this level of psychological distress was becoming apparent in 2020 and 2021, it was considerably less clear whether these problems were translating into increased rates of deliberate self-harm or suicide. While hospital presentations with self-harm declined during the first months of the pandemic, more extensive data collection and coroners' reports usually lag behind events, so the picture about self-harm was unclear for a long time. To an extent it remains uncertain today, not least because so many factors affect rates of self-harm and suicide that it can be difficult to separate out any single factor and identify its impact.

The survey of 195 psychiatrists by the College of Psychiatrists of Ireland in May and June 2020 found that 64 per cent of psychiatrists reported increased referrals for self-harm or suicidal ideation at that time compared to earlier in the pandemic.[25] There was also evidence of increased lethality of self-harm in at least one Irish hospital compared to before the pandemic.[26] Did this represent a significant shift in patterns of self-harm and suicide during Covid-19?

This issue is an important one, not least because suicide statistics prior to the pandemic gave reason for guarded optimism.[27] Between 1990 and 2016 the global rate of suicide declined by a third.[28] In addition, Ireland's rate was generally below the European average. In 2017 the overall rate of suicide in Ireland was the ninth lowest of thirty-three countries, although Ireland's rate among 15- to 19-year-olds was the thirteenth highest of thirty-one countries.[29] While the overall trend was downward, then, further progress was needed.

Prior to Covid-19, the global decline in suicide was one of the most dramatic public health shifts of our generation. While even one suicide is one too many, and there was clearly much more to be done, it finally seemed that positive change was not only possible but happening. Suicide was in decline. What did the pandemic do to this trend?

In March 2021, data from the US showed that suicide there fell by almost 6 per cent in 2020, in the midst of Covid-19.[30] This gave further cause for hope, and today most studies confirm that increased rates of distress during the pandemic have not translated into increased rates of suicide—at least not yet.[31] This suggests that, despite the anxieties, stresses and depressive symptoms felt by many, despite the loneliness, frustration and disconnection, rates of suicide remained steady or even declined in some places during the pandemic. Finally, some good news amidst the bad. We really are *much* stronger than we think.

The stability of suicide rates during Covid-19 might be attributable to a combination of better-than-expected coping and national suicide prevention policies in many countries. In Ireland, *Connecting for Life: Ireland's National Strategy to Reduce Suicide, 2015–2020* was launched in 2015 by Healthy Ireland, the Department of Health, the Health Service Executive and the National Office for Suicide Prevention.[32] This national plan involves preventive and awareness-raising activities with the population as a whole, supportive work with local communities and targeted approaches for priority groups. The strategy, which has been extended to 2024, proposes high-quality standards of practice across service delivery areas and—most importantly—an underpinning evaluation and research framework. We need this, regardless of prevailing trends in rates of self-harm and suicide. To repeat: even one suicide is one too many.

Approaches rooted outside core mental health services are vital for addressing self-harm and suicide: managing alcohol problems and other addictions, reducing homelessness, reforming the criminal justice system and improving social care.[33] These challenges extend well beyond the health sector because suicide is an all-of-society issue that requires an all-of-society response—just like Covid-19.

OCTOBER 2021

October derives its name from the Latin and Greek word ôctō, *meaning 'eight'. It was once the eighth month in the calendar of Romulus. Now the tenth month, October is International Walk to School Month and Black History Month in the United Kingdom. Henry Ward Beecher, a nineteenth-century American clergyman, speaker and slavery abolitionist, said that 'October is the opal month of the year. It is the month of glory, of ripeness. It is the picture-month.' Nathaniel Hawthorne agreed: 'There is no season when such pleasant and sunny spots may be lighted on, and produce so pleasant an effect on the feelings, as now in October'. Lucy Maud Montgomery, Canadian author of* Anne of Green Gables, *was similarly seized: 'I'm so glad I live in a world where there are Octobers'. Me too.*

In the 1840s, William Wilde wrote at length about the closing years of the life of Jonathan Swift (1667–1745), dean of St Patrick's Cathedral and author of *Gulliver's Travels* (1726).[34] Swift died in 1745 and left a generous bequest for the establishment of Ireland's first psychiatric hospital, St Patrick's, which opened in 1757 and continues today on its original site, near Dublin's Heuston Station.[35]

In his final years, Swift's health and state of mind deteriorated substantially. This is the period that interested Wilde. His writings obsess over Swift's final illness, the shape of Swift's skull and what the latter might reveal about the former. Wilde was not alone in this peculiar obsession.

Speculation about Swift's mental health was widespread and stemmed from the fact that in 1742, three years before his death, a writ, *de Lunatico Inquirendo*, was issued, declaring Swift 'a person of unsound mind and memory, and not capable of taking care of his person or fortune'.[36] This followed a petition from Swift's friends, consideration of medical evidence and a declaration by a jury. Owing to this event, the state of Swift's mind during his closing years became the subject of extensive speculation among such figures as Samuel Johnson, William Makepeace Thackeray and Sir Walter Scott, often many years after Swift's death.[37]

For Wilde, the most vexing suggestion was the idea that Swift became 'insane' towards the end of his life and was admitted to the very hospital that he funded. This was a clear impossibility, because Swift died in 1745 and St Patrick's opened in 1757, but rumours still swirled in Wilde's time, more than a century after Swift's death:

> It had been supposed by his biographers that a presentiment of his insanity induced [Swift] to devote his fortune to the erection of a lunatic asylum [and] that he was a fit inmate for his own asylum; it is generally believed that Swift was the first patient in the hospital, although it was not erected till several years after his death.[38]

Wilde was having none of it:

> Yet neither in his expressions, nor the tone of his writing, nor from an examination of any of his acts, have we been

as yet able to discover a single symptom of insanity, nor
aught but the effects of physical disease, and the natural
wearing and decay of a mind such as Swift's, hastened,
perhaps, by disappointed ambition, the bereavement of his
friends, public ingratitude, the want of those companions,
with tastes and habits suited to his own, with whom he
had so long enjoyed the most friendly intercourse, and the
collapse ensuing upon the retirement from those exciting
political, as well as literary matters, in which he had previously engaged.[39]

After studying contemporaneous accounts of Swift's symptoms, Wilde settled on Swift's stomach as the likely cause of
the great man's decline:

From the foregoing recital of his symptoms we learn that
whatever the real, original, exciting cause of Swift's bodily
ailment may have been, it is plain that it was attributed
both by himself and his physicians, to some derangement
of the stomach, and the remedies prescribed for him are
conclusive on this point.

It has been shown that these gastric attacks were, in early
life at least, induced by irregularities of diet. It is also evident
that they were attended with vertigo, deafness, sickness of
stomach, pain in the head, diminution of muscular power,
as shown by his tottering gait, and numbness or some slight
loss of sensation in the upper extremities.

That these in turn were symptomatic of some cerebral
affection is manifest; but how far it depended on, or was

induced by gastric disease, it is now difficult to determine; cases are, however, on record, which tend to show that all the early symptoms of [Swift's] malady may be produced by affections of the stomach and alimentary canal.

As Swift advanced in years his symptoms became more decidedly cerebral, and the attacks were induced by causes which acted more on the mental than the corporeal nature, such as excitements of various kinds, great mental labour, and strong emotions, to which the peculiarity of his disposition, and the position which he occupied, especially predisposed him.[40]

Swift made everything worse by being 'headstrong and unmanageable':

Swift certainly drank more wine, took more violent exercise, and was subjected to more frequent and stronger excitements, than a judicious physician of the present day would recommend, or could with safety permit; but then it must be remembered how very headstrong and unmanageable a patient he was, and also that he was, for the most part, his own medical adviser.[41]

This was Swift's character, not evidence of 'insanity'. Wilde is clear that Swift's communication problems 'arose either from paralysis of the muscles by which the mechanism of speech is produced, or from loss of memory of the things which he wished to express', as opposed to 'insanity or imbecility':

That the law appointed guardians of his person is no proof whatever of his insanity; for there are hundreds of cases in which the law very properly interferes with a man's estate, although he may not be either legally or physiologically insane, but simply incapable of managing his affairs; and it must be borne in mind that Swift had no family nor any near relatives, and scarcely a single friend, to look after him in his latter years.[42]

Swift lived just three years after guardians were appointed in 1742. He did not write during this period and lived in relative isolation. It now appears that Swift suffered from Ménière's Disease, a disorder of the inner ear that affects hearing and balance, and also causes vertigo and tinnitus.[43] Swift complained about these symptoms to his friend Alexander Pope in 1736, noting that he could no longer write, read or think clearly as a result.[44]

Swift also experienced memory loss, likely a result of cerebrovascular disease (impaired blood supply to the brain), which further reduced his mental abilities.[45] Consistent with this, Wilde reports that post-mortem examination of Swift's skull showed signs of cerebrovascular disease rather than anything else.[46] Wilde is surprised that Swift did not develop this condition earlier in life, in the light of the difficulties he faced:

We only wonder that Swift did not become deranged years previously; with a mind naturally irritable, a political intriguer, peevish and excitable; his ambition disappointed, his friendships rudely severed, his long-cherished hopes blighted; out-living all his friends, alone in the world, and witnessing the ingratitude of his country; while, at the same time, he laboured under a most fearful physical disease, in the very seat of reason, the effects of which were of the most stunning character, and serving in part to explain that moodiness and moroseness of disposition, which bodily infirmity will, undoubtedly, produce—we repeat, we only wonder that his mind did not long before give way.[47]

When Swift's mind eventually did 'give way', the immediate cause was cerebrovascular disease rather than 'insanity'. Despite this problem, or possibly because of it, Swift remained resolute that he would leave funds in his will to found an asylum for the mentally ill. Wilde points to Swift's long-term commitment to this idea, well prior to his decline and death in 1745:

It is evident that Swift had long entertained the idea of establishing such an institution; and so early as November, 1731, when he wrote the verses on his own death, we find his determination thus graphically described in the concluding stanza of that celebrated poem:

He gave the little wealth he had
To build a house for fools and mad;
And showed by one satiric touch,
No nation wanted it so much.[48]

St Patrick's, also known as 'Swift's Hospital', opened in 1757, twelve years after Swift's death. More than two and a half centuries later, this 'noble institution', as Wilde called it, still operates, as St Patrick's University Hospital, part of St Patrick's Mental Health Services.[49] During the Covid-19 pandemic, St Patrick's, like all similar facilities, had to adapt its model of service delivery, innovating to ensure continued care.[50]

In June and July 2021, the organisation's annual *Attitudes to Mental Health and Stigma Survey* reported a rise of 16 per cent in the number of people receiving mental health care, compared to 2019.[51] Clearly, the pandemic was having an effect not only on rates of anxiety and depressive symptoms but also on presentations for treatment, assistance and support. Consistent with this, the survey found that 56 per cent of respondents were more comfortable talking openly about their mental health in 2021 compared to before the pandemic.

People admitted to inpatient facilities for the treatment of mental illness faced particular problems during Covid-19. In March 2021, Drs Caitriona McCarrick, Andrew Gribben and Declan Lyons at St Patrick's pointed to the unique position of psychiatry inpatients during the pandemic.[52] For these patients, periods of leave from hospital are a key part of therapeutic care and recovery. Afternoons out with friends or staying overnight with family can be vital steps towards discharge from inpatient psychiatric care. Covid-19 restrictions made such leave difficult in many hospitals, and greatly reduced visits by family and friends. This was one of the many challenges generated by the pandemic in psychiatric facilities—difficulties with graded reintegration and phased discharge from inpatient care, just when it was needed most.

The pandemic also presented deep challenges to the mental well-being of hospital and healthcare workers around the world.[53] In the US, one study of 921 allied health professionals in April 2020 (early in the pandemic) found that 86 per cent reported feeling stressed with regard to changes in work environments and transmission of the virus.[54] This is not surprising: hospitals were challenging, uncertain places, especially at the start of the pandemic, as Seán O'Hagan pointed out in *The Observer*:

> Those most at risk of suffering post-traumatic stress are the frontline medical staff who, in the first chaotic weeks of the Covid-19 pandemic, may have felt overwhelmed by the dramatically increased levels of patient suffering and deaths, as well as at risk from infection from inadequate PPE [personal protective equipment] and anxious about bringing the virus home with them […] it may well be those we heralded as heroes who will be among the most vulnerable, alongside key workers on low incomes who also toiled through this long emergency at considerable and often unnecessary risk to their health, their lives.[55]

These problems were replicated in Ireland and around the globe.[56] In China, one study of 1,257 hospital healthcare workers in January and February 2020 found high levels of distress (72 per cent), symptoms of depression (50 per cent), anxiety (45 per cent) and insomnia (34 per cent).[57] These rates were substantially higher than those in the general population, reflecting the additional stresses of hospital work, especially in China. Risk factors for poor mental health included female gender, being a nurse and working on the front line. In some countries, healthcare workers faced violence from a frustrated public, further diminishing morale.[58]

In Ireland, a survey of 370 radiographers between March and May 2020 found that four in every ten reported burn-out symptoms owing to the pandemic, and three in ten considered changing jobs or retiring since it started.[59] The survey of 195 psychiatrists by the College of Psychiatrists of Ireland in May and June 2020 found that 61 per cent reported increased workloads; 46 per cent reported decreased well-being; and 51 per cent had diminished ability to avail of annual leave.[60]

Overall, it is now established that the rate of significant psychological distress among healthcare workers (approximately 40 per cent) was double that in the general population (approximately 20 per cent).[61] To remedy this during the pandemic and to prevent it in the future, healthcare staff require careful rostering (to distribute stresses fairly), ability to take leave (without placing colleagues under pressure), organisational support from employers (to prevent burn-out)[62] and, where necessary, 'psychological first aid' (to assist those who struggle).[63] These steps are essential to ensure that the understandable stresses of this or any future pandemic do not become lasting psychological problems.

There was also a need to manage the transition to on-line working with some care. The complexities of this shift were underlined in the survey by the College of Psychiatrists of Ireland, which indicated that a majority of psychiatrists 'felt they were ill equipped' for the change, with many experiencing connectivity problems.[64] This was certainly true for me: my home WiFi flickers from time to time, creating problems in interpreting subtle nuances of communication and, on occasion, difficulty in hearing people.

I realise that the movement to on-line services was essential, and might outlast the pandemic in certain circumstances, but mental health care is a very human endeavour. Interpersonal connections on-line are different from those in person. In 1978, journalist Bernard Levin wrote in *The Times* that 'the silicon chip will transform everything, except everything that matters, and the rest will still be up to us'.[65] Figuring out the strengths and weaknesses of on-line healthcare requires time and careful thought—both of which were challenging during the emergency phase of the pandemic.

The stress resulting from moving on-line amplified the responsibilities and anxieties experienced by many healthcare staff. Work cultures did not always help, especially in medicine, which has a grim culture of overwork, seemingly rooted in an assumption that postgraduate medical training is about endurance, survival and pain rather than knowledge, compassion and care. This is a long-standing problem that pre-dates the pandemic by several centuries.

When Wilde trained as a doctor in the 1830s, he was incessantly busy, serving as an apprentice to renowned surgeon Abraham Colles at Dr Steevens's Hospital in Dublin (beside St Patrick's); receiving tuition from surgeon James Cusack and physician Henry Marsh; and attending the school of anatomy, medicine and surgery in Park Street, before becoming a Licentiate of the Royal College of Surgeons in 1837. In addition to his writing and other activities, Wilde gained postgraduate training and experience in London and Vienna, and in 1844 opened his own hospital, St Mark's 'Ophthalmic Hospital and Dispensary for Diseases of the Eye and Ear' in Dublin, making for a life of frenzied activity and continuous work.[66] Deeply dedicated to his profession in the broadest sense, Wilde assumed additional duties over the following decades, including analysis of census figures about disability and disease, as well as his extraordinary, epic account of 'Cosmical Phenomena, Epizootics, Famines, and Pestilences' over the course of Irish history (Chapter 1).

Medicine has always demanded dedication, but this has too often translated into a tradition of overwork, a sense of responsibility for dysfunctional systems and excessively long shifts in hospitals.[67] I worked as a non-consultant hospital doctor (NCHD) in training posts around Ireland for many years after graduating as a doctor in 1996 and before becoming a consultant (specialist) in 2005. Hours were long: for a weekend 'on call', the NCHD would enter the hospital at 8 a.m. or 9 a.m. on Friday and remain at work in the hospital continuously until 6 p.m. on Monday. On a quiet weekend, the NCHD might get some sleep. On a busy weekend there would be no sleep at all. It was horrific and, from lunchtime Saturday until Monday morning, unpaid.

After staggering home on Monday evening, the NCHD was back at work at 8 a.m. or 9 a.m. on Tuesday, and each day thereafter. There was no time off following nights or weekends 'on call' in the hospital. Rosters were often 'one-in-three' or 'one-in-four', meaning that the NCHD was 'on call' in the hospital every third or fourth night, and every third or fourth weekend, in addition to working five days a week. Thinking back, it was clearly ludicrous, deeply inhumane and probably dangerous. It is a miracle that anyone survived, let alone remained in medicine.[i]

Today, the European Working Time Directive has made certain improvements and given NCHDs a day off after a night on call. Even so, NCHDs are still expected to work lengthy shifts that exceed safe limits.[68] When the stresses of Covid-19 were added in, the position of NCHDs and many other doctors around the world became untenable. As we have seen, many struggled. Most found a way to cope, but some, tragically, did not.[69]

The absence of compassion in our treatment of NCHDs is particularly distressing at a time when solidarity remains central to our efforts to address the Covid-19 pandemic and hold our societies together. Hopefully, appreciation of healthcare staff will be one legacy of this dreadful pandemic, recognising the sacrifices made by so many during the white

---

i   But we did, weirdly.

heat of the outbreak, when we relied on the steadiness of GPs, nurses, hospital doctors, testing-centre staff and many others to provide a bulwark against infection, illness, anxiety and despair. We owe them.

NOVEMBER 2021

November takes its name from the Latin word novem, *meaning 'nine', recalling a time when November was the ninth month of the year. November is National Novel Writing Month, when we are encouraged to write a 50,000-word manuscript.*[ii] *For Thoreau, 'the thinnest yellow light of November is more warming and exhilarating than any wine they tell of. The mite which November contributes becomes equal in value to the bounty of July.' D.H. Lawrence had a similar thought: 'Now in November nearer comes the sun down the abandoned heaven'. For Lucy Maud Montgomery, November is a liminal time, ripe with possibility: 'There is always a November space after the leaves have fallen when she felt it was almost indecent to intrude on the woods … for their glory terrestrial had departed and their glory celestial of spirit and purity and whiteness had not yet come upon them'.*

I stand outside the Village Coffee House in Templeogue and savour the best espresso in Dublin. Caffeine courses through me, leaving a bitter, exhilarated taste. My mind

---

ii   Everyone has a novel inside them. Mine is staying in there.

races, my soul shudders. Abruptly, everything makes sense: the arc of history, the meaning of life, the tender mercies of being. No need to understand; just experience—this moment, this life, this coffee. The mindfulness of the mindlessness of caffeine.

November is the greatest month: the promise of winter, untainted by Christmas, undiluted by signs of spring. Late autumn as it should be: unapologetic, cold. I love it.

The pandemic grinds on. A fourth wave emerges, leaving everyone demoralised by seemingly endless oceans of infection. Reopening society after the third wave did not go to plan: since last month, cases have risen across Europe.[70] In Ireland, daily case numbers now exceed 2,000; hospitalisations are increasing; intensive care beds fill up.[71]

Despite an adult immunisation rate that exceeds 90 per cent, Covid-19 is proving tireless. The Delta variant dealt a blow to hopes for a rapid end to this pandemic and was soon to be followed by Omicron. Commentators blame the government for perceived failings.[72] This month, I devour Richard Chambers's just-published book, *A State of Emergency: The Story of Ireland's Covid Crisis*, detailing how Ireland handled the pandemic from the beginning.[73] It is a gripping read. As I see it, our government handled the pandemic relatively well, all things considered. Our leaders performed better than I might have predicted; public health experts excelled.

In the past, some of our politicians have held fascinating views about health. Almost half a century ago, in 1978, Charles Haughey, Minister for Health and Social Welfare, outlined his assessment of the Irish and our prospects for physical and mental well-being:

> Theoretically, the job of maintaining and improving the health of this nation should be relatively easy. We are in a privileged position. We produce good food, our air is still fairly pure, our climate is temperate. There is space for all of us to move around. Even for those in the built-up areas, the countryside, the mountains, and the sea are within easy reach. Our temperament should be conducive to health. Our natural pace for doing things may not be regarded by the economists as ideal for the technological age, but it allows for a more civilised existence, a more human approach to one another and it creates less stress than one feels in other countries and larger centres of population. Our sense of humour too is another asset which should contribute to a healthy lifestyle.[74]

Despite these boons, including our sense of humour, Haughey saw problems:

> We have all these advantages over most countries in the Western world. Have we, therefore, any excuse for not being the healthiest nation in Europe, at least?
>
> Unfortunately, we are not.
>
> In fact, we suffer an amazing incidence of sickness for a nation of our size and circumstances. Our rate of hospital admissions, for instance, for physical and mental illness is abnormally high. Clearly, a new approach is called for.

Haughey was correct about Ireland's high rates of hospitalisation, but this is not necessarily evidence of increased illness because different countries use primary care services (e.g. GPs), specialist care (e.g. outpatient clinics) and hospital beds (for physical and mental ill health) very differently. Some countries have well-developed primary care and outpatient services, while others lean towards hospitals. Haughey placed Ireland firmly in the latter category.

This tendency towards hospitalisation was already known in relation to mental illness since the early 1970s and before. Irish psychiatrist Anthony Clare explored this theme in his dissertation for a master's degree in psychiatry (MPhil.) from the University of London in 1972.[75] His research centred on seventy-six patients from Ireland who made their first contact with the psychiatric services of the Camberwell area of London in 1970, and seventy-six patients from England, Scotland and Wales living in the same area. Clare found that psychiatric referral rates were higher among the Irish than among the indigenous population but that the rate of schizophrenia was not higher among Irish migrants, despite reportedly high rates of the condition in Ireland and among Irish migrants in the US.[76]

The idea that the Irish have an increased rate of mental illness was a long-standing one and, as Clare pointed out in his thesis, still prevalent in 1970s Ireland. It was to take several more decades of research and exploration to dismantle this notion of the 'mad Irish' and to prove definitively that the Irish do not have, and never had, a higher rate of mental illness than other people.[77] As far back as 1972, however, Clare showed that the Irish became engaged in specialist psychiatric care, as opposed to general practice care, at an earlier stage in their condition. This led to an apparently higher rate of illness and—in Ireland, at least—a higher rate of hospital usage compared to other countries. As Haughey pointed out six years later, rates of hospital admission for both mental and physical illness were 'abnormally high' in Ireland.

The precise meaning of rates of hospitalisation became topical again during Covid-19, when daily news bulletins led with numbers of new cases, hospitalisations and admissions to ICU. Suddenly, politicians were to the forefront of interpreting these statistics and making sweeping, unprecedented decisions based on them, restricting our liberty and reaching deep into our lives to minimise risks presented by the virus. Were our leaders reading the numbers correctly?

For the most part, yes. It is my view that our political and public health leaders reacted well to an unprecedented situation.[78] Like most people, they were unprepared and at times scrambled to stay abreast of developments. Despite this, I identified a willingness to both 'follow the science' (insofar as such a thing was possible) and make political judgements that were informed by medical advice but not completely governed by it. It was a tightrope act, so there were wobbles, but balance was achieved more often than not.

While future historians will provide a definitive assessment of the public health interventions chosen by our leaders, it is already clear that vaccines are performing precisely as predicted: they do not solve all our problems, but they are dramatically dampening the impact of the fourth wave. I see this around me every day in my clinical work. Jon Henley and Philip Oltermann made this point clearly in *The Observer* in mid-November 2021:

> Vaccine take-up on the continent is highest in southern Europe, with Portugal, Malta and Spain all having double-vaccinated more than 80% of their populations, and Italy not far behind on 73%, according to figures from Our World In Data. Seven-day rolling averages of new daily infections are the lowest in the bloc in those countries, at around 100 per million people—but they are edging up, and where vaccine take-up is low they have surged.[79]

These developments add enormously to the urgency of the vaccination booster campaign.[80] Vaccines save lives.

In this light, and writing as a psychiatrist, I cannot ignore the fact that people with pre-existing mental illness are at substantially increased risk of Covid-19 compared to people without mental illness, and urgently require vaccination and boosters. In the US, the odds of infection with Covid-19 are over seven times greater in people with depression or schizophrenia compared to the general population.[81] [iii] These are shocking statistics that make a diagnosis

---

iii This remains true even after taking account of other factors that might affect risk, including age and medical problems such as

of mental illness one of the largest single risk factors for contracting Covid-19.

There is every reason to believe that these US statistics also apply in Ireland. People with mental illness have always suffered systematic discrimination in health and social care in every country in which this has been examined, including Ireland. Health emergencies exacerbate the problem. As we have seen, the 1918 influenza pandemic (Spanish 'flu) hit Ireland's enormous, crowded psychiatric hospitals especially hard.[82] As a result, people who were deemed 'mentally ill' suffered far more than those who were mentally well, and were more likely to die.

Today, during Covid-19, our mental health services have improved and are, for the most part, based in the community, but people with mental illness are still at increased risk of neglect, homelessness, imprisonment and denial of rights.[83] Many have difficulties in accessing healthcare at the best of times, let alone during a pandemic. In 2019, prior to Covid-19, the Inspector of Mental Health Services, Dr Susan Finnerty, pointed out that 'patients with serious mental illness experience reduced access to health care either through delayed presentation, reduced uptake of health screening and preventive care, difficulty coping with the demands of monitoring and treatment, or misattribution of symptoms'.[84] Reduced access to public health

cancers, cardiovascular disease, type 2 diabetes, obesity, chronic kidney disease, chronic obstructive pulmonary disease, asthma and substance use disorders.

advice is, clearly, an especially urgent problem during a pandemic.

For this reason, community mental health teams need to be strengthened and supported to give people with mental illness improved access to both mental health care and public health advice. There are also calls to prioritise vaccination for people with severe mental illness in order to meet their health needs and help prevent adverse outcomes from the virus.[85] With this in mind, it is vital that services for the mentally ill are not only protected but enhanced during Covid-19.[86] Equity is essential at a time of national crisis, so we must ensure that people with mental illness and their families are not neglected, as they were in previous emergencies.

In addition to protecting mental health services and optimising vaccination rates into the future, social care has a role in minimising some of the other adverse effects of this seemingly endless pandemic. There has been an unprecedented shift in drinking patterns over the past two years, and this is linked to increased concerns about domestic violence, which is in turn complicated by restrictions on travel and other infection-reducing measures.[87] People with disabilities appear to be at particular risk of adverse outcomes during periods of restrictions, including violations of rights.[88]

All told, pre-existing disadvantages are exacerbated by the pandemic, long-standing injustices are made worse and those who have suffered in the past suffer more during Covid-19. Old problems are writ large, familiar patterns emerge.

The primary costs here are diminished well-being, increased mental ill health and worsening social problems. In May 2020, an independent research report by Simetrica-Jacobs and the London School of Economics and Political Science examined *The Wellbeing Costs of COVID-19 in the UK* and calculated an indicative monetary value for the total well-being cost of the pandemic to adults.[89] This cost came out as approximately £2.25 billion per day, or about £43 per adult per day. This is an interesting, important statistic but, as the report points out, there are other impacts too, which can be even more difficult to quantify. Newspapers are consistently full of warnings about increasing psychological problems among young people, mental health services under pressure and yet more suffering to come.[90] Looking at the news on any given day, one might be forgiven for despairing.

That would be a mistake. All of this bad news should be balanced against plentiful evidence of strength, resilience and adaptation seen during this pandemic.[91] Also, from the outset, organisations such as the World Health Organisation, the Centers for Disease Control and Prevention (in the US) and the Health Service Executive have provided solid mental health advice that has, in my experience, helped many.[92] As this fourth wave continues, the essentials remain important: focusing on what we can control (which is not always easy), identifying major and minor stressors in our lives (some might be preventable, especially the minor ones), noticing unhelpful thinking patterns (such as lingering on negative news) and seeing ourselves as part of a larger whole (which adds perspective).[93] These things matter and can help us get through the dark times.

Periods when public health restrictions intensify or are reintroduced present particular challenges, especially if they are seen as unfair or discriminating against certain groups, such as older adults.[94] But it is primarily the virus that is unfair, not the government or its policies. Covid-19 just doesn't care.

Social media exchanges about these developments can prove pernicious because so much of the material is driven by emotion, bias, prejudice and lies rather than facts.[95] Novelist Elif Shafak writes that we live in an age of too much information, less knowledge and, sadly, even less wisdom.[96] Too often, social media compound these problems. This is regrettable, because social media can do great good by providing timely information and facilitating supportive networks. In times of panic, however, the negatives tend to outweigh the positives, unless we limit our consumption of social media, think critically about what we read and refrain from amplifying false or misleading material within our information communities.

Values matter, especially as the Covid-19 situation deteriorates again this month (November 2021). From the start, President Michael D. Higgins emphasised the importance of 'solidarity, care, compassion and kindness' in these straitened circumstances:

> I have mentioned solidarity as an essential value guiding us as we proceed. We must acknowledge that breaches of

solidarity damage, and have damaged, social cohesion in combating Covid, but our righteous concerns must not be allowed to dislodge us from our common purpose—that of, by following the advice in relation to public health which we are determined to do out of good citizenship, we will, together, suppress the virus.

Invoking solidarity requires of us, of course, an understanding of the different kinds of vulnerability that there are, the differences, too, in capacities and circumstances. Understanding this is what enables the fine lines that might accompany the broad brushstrokes of the measures we are taking, to be drawn—drawn with sensitivity, as well as with risk taken into account.[97]

Higgins highlights the need for compassion and kindness, even in the face of complex risk:

'Compassion', I suggest, must be discernible in language as well as actions. The significance of small, low-risk gestures and processes that are part of the interactions of living for those in different categories needs to be recognised and respected [...] 'Kindness' is precious. What we communicate with each other, and how, must not be in any form of cold language that invokes fear, but rather one that conveys a warmth, one that reflects a shared concern for us all living and working together as citizens, seeking to exercise our responsibilities stretched to the best of our capacity from an ethic of good citizenship.

These principles of 'good citizenship' extend to all during the pandemic: the well and the ill, the vaccinated and the unvaccinated, the hopeful and those who falter. Epictetus, a Greek Stoic philosopher, held that 'difficulties are things that show a person what they are'. How we respond to other people's difficulties is, perhaps, the most telling sign of all.

Cases rise as November ends, bitterly.

4. WINTER 2021:
WORKING

'Good character is not formed in a week or a month. It is created little by little, day by day. Protracted and patient effort is needed to develop good character.'

—*Heraclitus*

*T*his chapter takes us from December 2021 to February 2022 and focuses on the idea of 'work'. Wilde worked ceaselessly: seeing patients, establishing a new clinic and then a hospital, writing papers and books, and participating in the Irish census. He seemed unable to stop working and, perhaps as a result, showed poor judgement in relation to one young patient, Mary Travers. A very public court case followed, in 1864. Over a century and a half later, Covid-19 brought enormous changes to workplaces and work identities in Ireland and elsewhere. These shifts were very apparent in healthcare and other front-line settings, but also occurred more generally, as many people worked from home or changed work practices in other ways. Work is the prism through which many of us *see our lives and value ourselves: the pandemic questioned this practice. Like Wilde, many people are prone to intensive work and overwork, but we are more than our occupations. Will this realisation be a lasting legacy of Covid-19—a deeper awareness of work–life balance? Or will we slip back into our old ways almost immediately? This chapter explores these themes, along with the emergence of 'long Covid', which brings psychological problems for many after the acute infection but can be treated over time. Also in this chapter: I drink a great deal of coffee, get very wet, go to Iceland and see an owl.*

DECEMBER 2021

December brings winter, the end of the calendar year, holidays for many and religious festivals around the world. Charles Dickens was full of praise for December: 'Of all the months of the year there is not a month one half so welcome to the young, or so full of happy associations, as the last month of the year'. Russian poet Zinaida Gippius saw December as a time of contradiction and drama: 'December's immaculate coldness feels warm. December feels like blood.' It is a month of cold and warmth, endings and celebrations. Aristotle saw contradiction and challenge in splendour: 'To be hot is the nature of fire and snow's nature is white'.

On 18 February 1904, patients from St Mark's Ophthalmic Hospital for Diseases of the Eye and Ear, founded by William Wilde in 1844, were transferred to the new Royal

Victoria Eye and Ear Hospital on Adelaide Road in Dublin. The impressive new red-brick building was constructed to house an amalgamation of Wilde's beloved hospital with the National Eye Hospital. This was a historic day, the culmination of a vision initially outlined by Wilde, who had died almost three decades earlier.

The Royal Victoria Eye and Ear Hospital still operates today, an iconic building set back from a busy road, in a secluded nook of its own. It has a quaint, old-world air from the outside, and retains a marble bust of Wilde on its main staircase. The bust is an appropriate memorial to a man whose energy and passions seemed to know no bounds, and whose interests in the human eye and ear were unending, resulting, ultimately, in this hospital (and much else besides). Wilde's legacy is everywhere.

Novelist Colm Tóibín writes about this ardent, over-active quality of Wilde in his 2018 book *Mad, Bad, Dangerous to Know: The Fathers of Wilde, Yeats and Joyce.*[1] He describes the great man's insatiable curiosity about people and the world, his appetite for company, his energy, his versatility and his endless desire for work. Wilde's labours included writing books and papers, ceaseless medical consultations and deep involvement in the Irish national census. As Roy Foster points out in a review, Wilde was the quintessential polymath—an eminent Victorian, a man of letters and, for much of his life, a very public figure.[2]

Wilde's career in medicine includes significant contributions to several fields. His work was especially notable in ophthalmology, the branch of medicine concerned with disorders of the eye. Following his training, in 1841 he opened a free dispensary for diseases of the eye and ear on Frederick Lane South, which was soon overwhelmed by demand.[3] In 1843 this service treated some 1,056 people, prompting Wilde to establish St Mark's 'Ophthalmic Hospital and Dispensary for Diseases of the Eye and Ear' in 1844, at 16 Mark Street. Clearly, there was substantial unmet need for diagnosis and treatment of ailments of the eye and ear in nineteenth-century Dublin. Wilde intended to fill that gap.

Wilde's enthusiasm for information and numbers was immediately apparent at the new hospital. St Mark's first annual report presented detailed statistics about its patients. In 1850 the hospital added statistics about all surgeries performed over the previous three years. The extensive list of operations includes cataract extractions and a range of other procedures. Also in 1850, the hospital moved to 32 Lincoln Place, in a further testament to Wilde's growing appetite for medical work and the endless need for care.

From a clinical point of view, Wilde was interested in all conditions of the eye, but had a particular fascination with trachoma, an infectious cause of blindness, which he had come across on his earlier travels in Egypt.[4] Trachoma was very common in Ireland in the latter part of the nineteenth century. Wilde's careful work on the condition contributed significantly to its decline, along with general improvements in diet and cleanliness.

Wilde made sure to provide clinical instruction at St Mark's from the start, for both established doctors and medical students. Widely known beyond Ireland, he communicated with fellow ophthalmologists overseas, many of whom came to Dublin to see him work. In 1851 he was visited by Albrecht von Graefe (1828–70), the famed German ophthalmologist, who watched him perform several operations.[5] Ten years later, Wilde sent his son, Henry Wilson, who was studying medicine, to visit von Graefe's clinic in Berlin. In 1853 Wilde was appointed Surgeon Oculist [eye doctor] to Her Majesty Queen Victoria.[6]

Perhaps the most interesting aspect of Wilde's ophthalmic work, however, comes not from his individual patient care or even the establishment of St Mark's but from his involvement in the Irish censuses of 1841, 1851, 1861 and 1871. While his epic, 270-page 'Table of Cosmical Phenomena, Epizootics, Famines, and Pestilences in Ireland' in the 1851 census is, perhaps, especially relevant in the era of Covid-19,[7] Wilde the ophthalmologist was in plentiful evidence throughout the census reports too. More specifically, Wilde presented detailed data about the prevalence of blindness in nineteenth-century Ireland, and thus brought much-needed attention to the parlous situation of the blind at the time.[8]

In 1851 Wilde reported that there were 7,587 blind people in Ireland, of whom 12 per cent resided in workhouses, meaning that most lived at home and were cared for by their families.[9] At that point, there were 270 places available in institutions for the blind in Ireland. Wilde challenged the notion, prevalent at the time, that any blind person over the age of 22 years could not be trained. He believed that the government should make further provision for them to earn their living. As usual, he supported his position with numbers, details and statistics, drawn largely from his beloved census.

Wilde also drew attention to the deaf, reporting that there were (in the language of the times) 4,747 'true deaf and dumb' people among the Irish population of 6,552,386 in 1851.[10] This amounted to one deaf and dumb person per 1,380 people in the general population, which was quite similar to Europe more broadly (estimated at one case per 1,593). Wilde, as ever, provided nuanced historical information to supplement and contextualise his statistics:

> It was believed in ancient times, and the idea is still entertained in other countries less favoured than our own, that the deaf and dumb are incapable of improvement or instruction of any kind [...]
>
> It is remarkable that the forms and complications of mutism observed in the present day are precisely similar to those described as existing in Judea nearly nineteen hundred years ago—the deaf and dumb; the lunatic deaf and dumb, or those possessed with a spirit; the blind and dumb; and the partially deaf and dumb. Of the latter form, an instance is related by St Mark, of 'one who was deaf, and had an impediment in his speech', and of whom it is said that, when the miracle of the Saviour was performed, 'his ears were opened, and the string of his tongue was loosed, and he *spake plain*'.
>
> It remained, however, for the enlightenment and benevolence of modern times to achieve the task of systematically

elevating this unhappy class to the level of ordinary humanity, by kindness, judicious training, and ingeniously devised
instruction.[II]

After Wilde the statistician and Wilde the historian had
said their pieces about the prevalence and history of
deafness, Wilde the medical scientist emerged, seeking
to establish whether, and to what degree, deafness was
inherited. Enquiring further into the numbers, Wilde
reported that in seventy-seven marriages between a hearing person and a deaf person there was one deaf child out
of 182 children.[12] This was twice the rate of deafness in the
general population. In five marriages between two deaf
people, one of fourteen children was deaf, which was one
hundred times the rate in the general population. These
findings were consistent with a genetic element in risk of
deafness.

Ultimately, however, it was Wilde the social reformer
who had the most to say about the position of the 'deaf and
dumb' in nineteenth-century Ireland:

In any inquiry into the condition of the deaf and dumb,
two great objects present—a physiological and a social.
Under the former the deaf mute may be classed among
those afflicted with permanent disease, either congenital or
acquired, and, as such, demands the careful investigation
of the statistician; and all the causes and phenomena of the
affection solicit attention equally with those circumstances
attendant upon lunacy, idiocy, blindness, or any of the

other persistent maladies which affect certain portions of the community in all countries.

Under the latter head, the deaf mute claims the special attention of the philanthropist, and the protection of the State, owing to the forlorn condition to which he is reduced by his affliction, the difficulty he experiences in expressing his wants, and his inability either to educate himself, or to receive instruction through the ordinary channels.[13]

All told, Wilde used the census to draw public and professional attention to the plight of the 'deaf and dumb' throughout Ireland. This was consistent with his own clinical work and his long-standing interest in providing medical care to the poor, the disadvantaged and people with disabilities, of whom, he established, there were many more than was commonly acknowledged. Their problems were substantial and needed to be addressed.

Interestingly, Wilde concluded his consideration of the 'deaf and dumb' by discussing 'some of the questions which, in a legal point of view, affect the deaf and dumb', including their roles as witnesses in court.[14] This focus was consistent with his broader interest in medico-legal matters throughout his career, which resulted in significant involvements in medico-legal cases at various points.[15] This activity attracted mixed attention, but it accurately reflected Wilde's preoccupation with both the development of medical knowledge and its application in different areas of life. He was a realist, keen to make things happen both inside and outside the clinic.

In this spirit, Wilde was never afraid to step outside the consulting room and get involved in discussions and debates beyond the world of medicine—even if this meant becoming embroiled in complex legal cases. Ultimately, it was all grist to his mill. Wilde's appetite for engagement knew no limits. He literally could not stop.

As if all of these activities and involvements were not enough, Wilde became editor of the *Dublin Quarterly Journal of Medical Science* in the mid-1840s.[16] Characteristically, he started his new role in grand style with a forty-eight-page 'editor's preface' in the February 1846 issue, detailing 'the history of periodic medical literature in Ireland, including notices of the medical and philosophical societies of Dublin'.[17] This was Wilde at his most assured, on home ground, drawing history and medicine together to summarise the past and set a chart for his new role as editor.

Over the following years, Wilde's application and attention to detail were extraordinary, not least in his own papers detailing his survey of Irish doctors on the subject of Famine diseases, in late August 1848.[18] His lengthy accounts of 'epidemic fever' during this period resonate strongly with the current pandemic: infection is eternal, medicine is social, and we never lack for problems or—if we look with care—solutions. It's all here.

Ever restless, Wilde wrote biographies of leading figures in Irish medical history, including Bartholomew Mosse (founder of the Rotunda Hospital), Thomas Molyneux (president of the King and Queen's College of Physicians in Ireland) and Robert Graves (one of Ireland's most celebrated medics).[19] Wilde's name now belongs on this list of luminaries.

Wilde did not limit his biographical writing to doctors and, in the 1870s, wrote extensively about Gabriel Beranger (1725–1817), a Dutch artist with an interest in Irish antiquities, in the *Journal of the Royal Historical and Archaeological Association of Ireland*.[20] His *Memoir of Gabriel Beranger and His Labours in the Cause of Irish Art and Antiquities from 1760 to 1780* was completed by Lady Wilde following his death in 1876, and published in book form in 1880.[21]

In this memoir, Wilde makes an interesting point about biographical writing, which appears relevant to the task of the present book, looking at Wilde's life and work in the context of Covid-19:

> Every biographer who wishes to be impartial should, for the occasion at least, live among the scenes and during the period when and where the personage whose character he is limning resided. He ought to be well acquainted with the subject he has undertaken to describe, and, as far as possible, honestly identify himself with the pursuits, and exercise a fair critical discretion in reviewing the labours of the person who, for the time being, has become the chief actor in his drama.[22]

I am not entirely certain where the limits of 'fair critical discretion' lie with Wilde's own story, but I imagine that the Mary Travers case comes well within the reasonable boundaries of any account of his life. The Travers case was certainly the subject of much attention when it occurred in 1864 and no examination of Wilde's story is complete without it.

Mary Travers became a patient of Wilde's in 1854 when she was 18 years of age and he was 39.[23] Ten years later, shortly after Wilde received his knighthood in 1864, Travers began to hint that he had given her chloroform and raped her two years earlier. She sent letters to newspapers intimating that this had occurred, and wrote a highly suggestive pamphlet about 'Dr and Mrs Quilp', who were clearly Wilde and Lady Wilde.

Lady Wilde was outraged and sent a letter to Travers's father, who was professor of medical jurisprudence at Trinity College. She informed the professor that his daughter was making unfounded allegations against her husband. Mary Travers came across the letter in her father's papers and sued Lady Wilde for libel, alleging that Wilde had indeed raped her in 1862. In court, Lady Wilde described the whole episode as 'fabrication' and sought to have it dismissed out of hand.

The judge, for his part, noted that Travers had not reported the alleged incident at the time and continued to attend public events with Wilde. In the end, the jury upheld the charge of libel against Lady Wilde. They awarded just one farthing in damages to Travers, but Wilde had to pay over £2,000 in legal costs—a substantial sum at the time.

The entire episode did not reflect well on Wilde. He did not take the stand at the trial, being under no legal obligation to do so. Even so, his failure to clarify the matter beyond doubt was seen as suggestive. He could have done more if he wished, but it appears that he did not want to provide precise details about his relationship with Travers. This is comprehensible, if dishonourable: his behaviour towards Travers was, at best, ill-judged and possibly worse. Their relationship is worth tracing over time, if only to highlight a blind spot in Wilde's conduct.

Wilde's association with Travers began when she became a patient of his in 1854, but it soon developed into some sort of friendship. Over time, the pair grew closer: Travers accompanied Wilde to public events; Wilde gave her money for clothes; Lady Wilde invited Travers for Christmas dinner; and, in 1862, Wilde, possibly keen to end the relationship at this stage, paid for Travers's fare to Australia.[24] Twice Travers set off for Australia and twice she turned back at Liverpool.

Travers was clearly ambivalent about leaving, but also found it difficult to stay. She called often to the Wildes' home at 1 Merrion Square during this period. On one such visit, Lady Wilde asked her whether she was trying to steal her husband. On another occasion, Travers reportedly entered Lady Wilde's bedroom uninvited, resulting in Travers rushing from the house.[25] Clearly, there was a crisis on the way.

From this point on, Travers's relationship with the Wildes deteriorated rapidly. She began to self-harm. At one point, she went into Wilde's consulting room and drank a bottle of laudanum in front of him, compelling him to accompany her to a pharmacy for the antidote, which he ensured that she took.

Matters escalated and Travers soon began to hint publicly that Wilde had raped her. In her pamphlet about 'Dr and Mrs Quilp', she accuses Dr Quilp of giving chloroform to a patient in order to have sex with her. She was clearly referring to Wilde.

Unable to tolerate continual public hints of this nature, Lady Wilde wrote to Travers's father about his daughter's 'disreputable conduct', in the letter that duly triggered the libel case:

Sir,

You may not be aware of the disreputable conduct of your daughter at Bray, where she consorts with all the low newspaper boys in the place, employing them to disseminate offensive placards, in which my name is given, and also tracts in which she makes it appear that she has had an intrigue with Sir William Wilde. If she chooses to disgrace herself, that is not my affair; but as her object in insulting me is the hope of extorting money, for which she has several times applied to Sir William Wilde, with threats of more annoyance if not given, I think it right to inform you that no threat or additional insult shall ever extort money for her from our hands. The wages of disgrace she has so basely treated for and demanded shall never be given to her.

Jane F. Wilde

After the jury found in favour of Travers, Lady Wilde described her as 'half mad', but the proceedings had already done considerable damage.[26] While much of the medical

profession supported Wilde, there was substantial coverage in the popular press and his public reputation was
tarnished.[27] All told, it was a remarkable, regrettable episode
that did not reflect well on Wilde, if only for his lack of
judgement in his relationship with Travers, who was, after
all, his patient.

The full truth of the Travers matter will likely never be
known, and it remains a fact that Travers won her libel case
against Lady Wilde. In 1865 Travers took a second libel case,
this time against *Saunders's News-Letter*, for suggesting that
she concocted a story about Wilde and committed perjury.
The jury threw that case out after just 25 minutes. Travers
took no further action. She died in 1919.

Wilde's medical career and various other involvements
continued after the case, but the episode took a toll on
him. For a man with such a keen understanding of so many
aspects of human life, the version of Wilde that emerged
during the trial was significantly less than flattering.

Today, almost 160 years after the libel case, as December
2021 comes to an end, I decide to visit the Royal Victoria
Eye and Ear Hospital to see the marble bust of Wilde.
Despite his flaws, he remains a figure of fascination for
many—including me.

I try to wander into the hospital one evening but am—reasonably and politely—stopped by security staff. I am advised
to come back another day when I have made an appointment.
This I do, and I access the building sometime later.

The bust of Wilde sits quietly in a windowsill on a busy
staircase in a bustling hospital. He is in pensive pose, head

back, eyes raised. I wonder what he is thinking about: his medical work, the Irish census, some obscure aspect of history, or possibly Mary Travers? I will never know.

I leave the hospital and walk along Adelaide Road. The evening is chilly. A fox runs across the street, slips through a fence and vanishes into some bushes. Soon I, too, go home.

JANUARY 2022

January rolls around. It is midwinter and the start of a new year. Many people find this a difficult month, the festivities of December firmly in the past and no holiday on the horizon. Even so, few can resist the idea of a new start, taking steps towards a better life. Essayist Charles Lamb wrote that 'no one ever regarded the first of January with indifference'. According to G.K. Chesterton, 'the object of a new year is not that we should have a new year. It is that we should have a new soul.' The pressure is substantial: we are expected to renew, refresh, rebuild and 'have a new soul'. Surely that is too much to ask, even of the most hardened optimist? And in the time of Covid-19 to boot?

It is January 2022. We are close on two years since this all began, and the pandemic is still happening. My hardened optimism is a little shaky. I need coffee.

I have profound sympathy for people who lack sympathy for coffee enthusiasts. I can think of few things more irritating than coffee aficionados who harp on endlessly about body, balance, blends and baristas. I am not alone in my concerns; many others feel likewise.[28] It is a disease of modernism.

There is profound hypocrisy in my stance, because the Covid-19 pandemic has seen me return to espresso-drinking with gusto. Right now, as I type these words, I am perched on an excruciatingly uncomfortable high stool with no back outside a hipster coffee 'venue' in Dublin's city centre. It is raining, so everyone who is seated outside is getting very, very wet. I pretend not to care because everyone else pretends not to care. We all care.[29]

The situation is even grimmer than it sounds. I am surrounded by men with manicured facial hair, clipped beards and carefully frayed woollen jumpers. There is nothing quiet about this desperation. We are all at the end of our tethers. And now we are sodden too, dripping rainwater onto our laptops. The scene is absurd, the ritual ridiculous, the players senseless.

I could go on about this experience in more detail and, like all obsessives after two espressos, I will.

The coffee-shop is a grotesque parody of itself, a baroque overstatement of all that is objectionable in *nouveau* coffee culture. Individually crafted chocolate brownies sit on tiny wooden pedestals, ethereal in their beauty but each scarcely more than a mouthful. Staff chat among themselves, inaccessible in their self-absorption. They work hard to look scruffy, but I know a thing or two about genuine scruff. This is not it. This is carelessness, curated.[i]

i   Give me strength.

The set-up is preposterous, the coffee mediocre, the prices indefensible. Yet here I am, addicted to these bizarre environments, unable to face the bitter, caffeinated, pulse-quickening truth: I have become one of *them*. These are now my people.

I blame Covid-19. Before the pandemic, I stayed away from coffee for several years. Now, after two years of restrictions and lockdowns, I am dependent on two double espressos each morning. This is a problem. Or is it?

Today I read (again) about the Japanese idea of *wabi-sabi*, which is the acceptance of imperfection and transience in life.[30] Nothing is perfect, nothing is complete, nothing lasts forever—and yet everything is beautiful if we accept things as they are.

A good espresso fits this paradigm with satisfying snugness: it is never perfect, it lasts just a few moments, it leaves me wanting more, and it is beautiful in a strange, transient, mysterious way. The Zen of coffee, the mindful macchiato, Buddha as barista.

The rain stops. I thrust coffee from my mind and return to the topic that occupies me as 2022 begins: the idea of 'long Covid' and what it might mean after the pandemic ends—if it ever really does. Wilde worried endlessly about the impact of infections. Living in a world of Covid-19, and working in a hospital, I do too. I read in today's *Financial Times* that millions of people have persistent symptoms of Covid-19 for as long as twelve weeks after being diagnosed with the infection.[31] Common issues include fatigue and breathing problems.

Hugely expensive 'treatments' have emerged on well-being websites and in high-end clinics around the world: vitamins, massages and elaborate retreats.[32] Most of this sounds like generic feel-good therapy, which can be helpful in its way but is not especially focused on Covid-19 or long Covid, which is now said to affect 114,000 people or more in Ireland.[33] If long Covid really turns out to be such a widespread problem, will we ever be able to say that the pandemic is truly over?

The idea that certain viruses can have lingering effects is not new and has been recognised with Covid-19 for some time.[34] The term 'long Covid' evolved over the past two years to describe signs and symptoms that continue or develop after acute infection with Covid-19. It includes ongoing symptomatic Covid-19 (from four to twelve weeks) and post-Covid-19 syndrome (twelve weeks or more), according to consensus recommendations published in November 2021.[35]

What this means is that the effects of Covid-19 infection can be prolonged in certain people and can continue for months in some cases.[36] Common persistent symptoms include fatigue, shortness of breath, joint pain, chest pain and diminished quality of life. It is clear that for many patients these lingering effects of the virus are substantial, disabling and persistent. But how many people are affected? How big is this problem, really?

At this point, as 2022 begins, more than 250 million people around the world have been infected with Covid-19. Over five million have died. These numbers are likely to be underestimates, owing to difficulties with diagnosis in many places, suboptimal health services in certain parts of the world and uneven reporting systems. Future research is likely to determine that the true incidence of Covid-19 was significantly higher.[37]

Even based on the figures we have today, however, it is clear that hundreds of millions of people around the world are at risk of long Covid after the acute pandemic ends. The implications for public health are substantial. The prominence of psychological and psychiatric symptoms as part of this syndrome suggests that the consequences for public *mental health* will form an especially challenging part of the work ahead.[38] With this in mind, it is important to establish precisely how common long Covid is, in order to estimate future healthcare need.[39] What does the research tell us so far?

In 2021, one group of Spanish researchers followed up 277 Covid-19 patients and identified symptoms of long Covid in just over half of them between ten and fourteen weeks after they first got the infection.[40] Fortunately, most symptoms were not too severe. Changes on X-rays and breathing tests appeared in less than 25 per cent of patients and also tended to be mild. Even so, over one third of these Covid-19 patients experienced fatigue many weeks after being infected, and two thirds of those with long Covid reported diminished quality of life. Clearly, this is a syndrome with significant impact on recovery among many people who would hope to have left Covid-19 far behind them after the acute infection.

The problem with long Covid is that some of its symptoms are quite vague. Many people are fatigued anyway, and almost everyone felt a dip in quality of life during the pandemic. What makes these symptoms different in long Covid?

One of the key features of long Covid is the *persistence* of symptoms such as fatigue, which is often combined with other, more specific problems, including impairments of taste and smell. These limitations have a much bigger impact than we might predict. Fatigue appears especially pernicious with long Covid: pervasive lack of energy, diminished capacity to initiate activity and a failure to feel refreshed after periods of rest. Being tired is tiring.

An inability to smell or taste food hugely diminishes quality of life. The UK's National Health Service advises that approximately one in ten cases of smell and taste problems persist after the initial Covid-19 infection is otherwise resolved, although many sufferers will see their sense of smell recover over time.[41] We know from other viruses that smell can return quite quickly in some people, within a couple of weeks, but in others it can take several months or longer to resolve. This is a substantial problem for many people.

Long Covid also has an extensive psychological dimension, in addition to fatigue and physical symptoms. For some sufferers, signs of poor mental health are apparent from the earliest stages after the acute infection. Studies conducted two weeks or more after physical recovery from Covid-19 detect high levels of anxiety (22 per cent), depression (21 per cent) and post-traumatic stress disorder (20 per cent).[42] This means that more than one patient in every five has specific psychological and psychiatric problems after 'recovery' from their initial Covid-19 infection. Given that more than 250 million people around the world have been infected to date, these numbers get very big very fast.

To compound matters, not only do more than one third of Covid-19 survivors report psychological distress but a similar proportion have sleep disorders. Sleep is essential for physical health, mental well-being and happiness.[43] Shakespeare described sleep as the 'chief nourisher in life's feast' and he was right. All too often, it seems that long Covid disrupts this vital function in people who have otherwise recovered from the infection. This is a double blow to those who suffered acute Covid-19 and expected to feel much better by now. For some, it feels as if Covid-19 will never end.

This anxiety is understandable. While many viruses produce 'long' syndromes and psychological after-effects, these problems appear to be more common among survivors of Covid-19 than survivors of certain other infections. Rates of anxiety and depression following Ebola, for example, are 14 per cent and 15 per cent respectively, compared to 22 per cent and 21 per cent with Covid-19. It is not entirely clear why Covid-19 is especially corrosive of mental health, but it is.

To complicate the picture even further, these problems are not equally distributed among Covid-19 patients, and they tend to persist.

In the first six months after infection with Covid-19, one third of all patients have a psychiatric or neurological diagnosis, but this increases to almost half (46 per cent) of those who were admitted to intensive therapy units.[44] Anxiety disorders, in particular, are present in 17 per cent of all Covid-19 patients during this period, but in 19 per cent of those admitted to intensive therapy units. Again, these problems seem to be more common following Covid-19 than other infections, especially among people with more severe illness. In addition, the risk of psychosis (severe mental illness involving some loss of contact with reality) is twice as high after Covid-19 as it is after influenza ('flu).

All of this paints a deeply concerning picture, as the data consistently show that Covid-19 presents a particular risk to mental health, even in its aftermath.[45] What can be done?

The first step in responding to long Covid is to try to prevent its occurrence in the first place. The existence of this condition underscores yet again the importance of adhering to public health guidance, promoting vaccination and supporting good general health in order to minimise the overall impact of Covid-19, including long Covid. Prompt diagnosis and treatment of Covid-19 are also likely to help. The basics still matter and will hopefully prevent more people being at risk of long Covid into the future.

The second step is to maintain a sense of perspective. The Covid-19 pandemic has not triggered a pandemic of mental illness. Covid-19 and the public health restrictions that it necessitated generated emotional challenges, diminished psychological well-being for some people, increased the likelihood of relapse in people with pre-existing psychiatric conditions and amplified the risk of new mental illness in certain groups, including people with severe Covid-19 infection and long Covid.

But these are problems, not a pandemic, and problems have solutions. There is no tsunami of mental illness owing to the pandemic, or owing to the public health measures it triggered, or owing to long Covid, or owing to any other reason. There are challenges, yes, but these are no reason to panic. As societies, we can handle this.

The third step is to realise that this problem is not entirely new. Most health professionals are already familiar with different post-viral syndromes that affect our patients after other infections, such as severe 'flu. Therefore, while the mental health consequences of Covid-19 appear especially common, they are not entirely novel.

Indeed, for many people, Covid-19 triggered a relapse of an existing mental illness rather than a new diagnosis. One especially large study of electronic case records in the US found that the incidence of any psychiatric diagnosis in the fourteen to ninety days after Covid-19 diagnosis was 18 per cent, including 6 per cent that were a first diagnosis.[46] For 12 per cent of Covid-19 patients, then, the virus triggered a relapse of an existing psychiatric condition rather than a new diagnosis. This highlights the importance of supporting people with pre-existing mental illness during the pandemic in order to prevent a worsening of their condition or full relapse. This is a predictable risk and, as such, should be more manageable.

The fourth step is to identify long Covid symptoms as early as possible and provide appropriate multi-disciplinary care. There is still very little evidence about the usefulness of specific psychiatric treatments following Covid-19, but the usual principles of mental health care will clearly apply, supplemented by good medical services in general practice and specialist clinics in our hospitals. Experience with similar post-viral syndromes will help, along with a willingness to learn about the new condition.[47]

Finally, we need more data. Follow-up studies are essential to better understand long Covid, calculate its incidence, estimate public health impact and—hopefully—identify specific treatments that work best. The need for reliable information about a new disorder has never been greater. Now that this condition is recognised, more information can be gathered and hopefully used to relieve the suffering of so many people for whom Covid-19 now feels like a chronic illness rather than an acute infection.[48] They need our support.

Despite these rather depressing statistics, the apparent endlessness of this pandemic and my escalating dependence on coffee, this month (January 2022) brings extraordinary shifts in the pattern of Covid-19 around the world, and real hope for the future.

At the start of January, the *Economist* reports that the Omicron variant, although spreading fast, causes a less severe illness.[49] In all corners of the globe, policies are being reconsidered in the light of the new situation. In China a 'zero Covid' policy still pertains, but, according to *The*

Observer, this approach is increasingly at odds with many other countries:

> The rest of the world is learning, slowly and with some difficulty, to live with Covid-19, but in China, authorities are doubling down on their 'zero-Covid' policy: trying to stamp out the disease [...]
>
> A key aspect of the policy is border closures. Few people are allowed in or out of China, and those who do enter the country face up [to] three weeks of government-enforced quarantine. Some other countries locked the world out for over a year in a bid to lock out the pandemic. But in 2022, Beijing is treading an increasingly solitary path.[50]

Here in Ireland, this month brings dramatic change in precisely the opposite direction. On 21 January, Taoiseach Micheál Martin addresses the nation, with bracing good news:

> Our journey through the pandemic has brought many twists and turns, and I have stood here and spoken to you on some very dark days. But today is a good day.
>
> Earlier, my government colleagues and I met to consider the latest report from the National Public Health Emergency Team. That report confirmed that we have weathered the Omicron storm. It confirmed that the rate of infection is reducing, and that all of the key indicators on which we base our decisions have stabilised and are going in the right direction. It confirmed that Ireland's world-

class vaccination programme and the roll-out of boosters has utterly transformed our situation. […]

Based on this evidence, we've concluded that the rationale and justification for continuing most of our public health restrictions are no longer in place. Therefore, from 6 a.m. tomorrow morning, the majority of public health measures that we have had to live with, will be removed.[51]

Just like that, everything changes. Martin leaves us in no doubt about the importance of vaccines in making today possible, but adds that 'the pandemic isn't over':

It will still require all of us to be vigilant. The changes we are making will likely lead to a temporary rise in infections in the short term, but we are advised that the impact of this rise will be limited by the scale of vaccination in the population.

With some understatement, the Taoiseach concludes that 'today is a good day':

… we should all take a moment to appreciate how far we've come; to appreciate the effort and sacrifice of those who put themselves in harm's way to keep us safe; to remember and appreciate the lives and contribution of those we lost. […]

Today's news will be warmly welcomed by many, but I'm conscious that some among us, including our more vulnerable, will be feeling some anxiety about re-engaging with others. For those who do feel like that, I'd ask you to be open about it, share it. We all need to be open with each other, be supportive of each other.

The following morning, the great majority of public health restrictions vanish with the dawn. Further relaxation is planned for the months ahead. The *Irish Times* front page summarises crisply: 'Emergency over'.[52] The *Irish Independent* announces 'A new beginning'.[53]

FEBRUARY 2022

If January is a cold month, burdened with righteous expectation, February is a time of realism: resolutions faded, December a distant memory, the new year under way. American poet William Cullen Bryant felt hope at this time of year: 'The February sunshine steeps your boughs and tints the buds and swells the leaves within'. Evenings lengthen. Light lasts longer. February is the shortest month, and it brings Saint Valentine's Day. Valentine was a third-century Roman clergyman who was martyred and buried on 14 February around the year 269. Celebrated since 496, his feast-day is now associated with love, a link well suited to February, with its intimation of brighter days ahead. Martin Luther King said that 'darkness cannot drive out darkness; only light can do that. Hate cannot drive out hate; only love can do that.' February brings light and love.

February starts much as January did, with me sitting in the rain outside a minimalist coffee-shop. Today the mood is better, the rain is lighter (it never stops) and Covid-19 restrictions are largely lifted. I order a celebratory espresso and pay a preposterous amount for a tiny cookie which is, in fairness, fabulous.

The sudden easing of restrictions has had significant impact, although reactions vary. Some people are simply delighted to see the end of the measures.[54] Many can barely wait to rip off their face-coverings at the first moment feasible.[55] Others are more circumspect, preferring to wait and see how things go. I belong to the latter camp: the suffering I saw among Covid-19 patients at work makes me cautious, if still optimistic, about this phase of the pandemic. *Festina lente*, hasten slowly, and all shall be well.

Few people are entirely unmoved by recent developments: there is a palpable sense of change. Are we finally closer to a post-Covid world? Or, at least, nearer to a life that is no longer dominated by restrictions, case numbers and worries about infection? Is such a thing even possible any more? Have some of us lost the ability to imagine it?

This month, my life divides crisply into two very different worlds: (a) work and (b) everything else.

I work in a psychiatry inpatient unit at a hospital and in an outpatient mental health service in a separate clinic building. In both settings, face-coverings remain mandatory and all Covid-19 restrictions remain in place. Healthcare locations are deemed high-risk, so full precautions still apply. In truth, most healthcare workers have seen such illness and suffering over the past two years that there is little appetite for easing restrictions at work. Many of the patients who attend us have pre-existing conditions and require additional protection, even now. Caution is appropriate. This is not over yet.

The nature of medical work has changed considerably over the past two years in hospitals, clinics, GP surgeries, nursing homes, Covid-19 testing centres and the various other locations where health and social care are provided. It has been a time of extraordinary transformation, with tele-medicine, e-consultations, flexible hours, shift-working, task-sharing and all manner of other innovations. Much of this has been good. Some did not work out.

I have seen positive changes myself every day since the start of the pandemic, in all my work locations. Since early 2020, the co-operation and flexibility that I witnessed across our health services are like nothing I have seen before. It has been breath-taking.[56]

I saw thousands of healthcare workers learn new skills, take on additional roles and step (carefully) towards risk rather than shrink from it. Public health teams reached out to communities and developed new ways of working that would be unimaginable at any other time. In many countries, including Ireland, testing and vaccination centres were staffed and opened in record time. New techniques were learned in the morning and applied in the afternoon.

Today, as the crisis subsides, I still see family doctors, primary care nurses and GP surgery receptionists adapt to ever-evolving guidelines, offer reassurance along with health advice, and guide the ill and worried to the best possible care—and to vaccination.

I see nurses arrive to work at the hospital, gown up into their uniforms and do their jobs with profound professionalism and unstinting dedication, even under trying circumstances. Shifts are moved around, people stay late, staff support each other.

Doctors at all levels of training provide increasingly complex care, navigate new clinical dilemmas and work with more heart and compassion than I have ever witnessed. Those who work in intensive care deserve special mention: doctors, nurses, physiotherapists, allied health professionals, catering staff, cleaners, orderlies, porters, chaplains and countless others. They all need each other, and we all need them, even now, as many people start to feel that the pandemic is almost over.[57] Covid-19 is far from finished with us, but it has eased.

For each of these healthcare workers there is a family at home, waiting. They are worried that Mum is overworking and stressed and does not take time off. They are worried that Dad opted for another extra shift at the weekend. They are worried that their partner—a speech and language therapist, nurse or social worker—is working all the hours in the week. Or that their daughter—a surgeon, manager or hospital porter—stays late every night, providing essential support and advice to the ill, the anxious and, tragically, the bereaved. All of this matters deeply, even now, as the situation improves.

Health service managers, too, have delivered in spades: late-night conference calls to resolve staffing rotas, finding resources to free up beds, providing supports to ensure that care is delivered where and when it is needed. These are difficult tasks, and all the more so in a pandemic. The chief executive officers of our hospitals have worked through long, hard nights to keep the whole operation on the road. They might not be the traditional face of front-line care but awesome responsibility rests on their shoulders, now more than ever. They still stay up late. This is not over yet.

Then there is the public, trying to navigate a path through this wretched pandemic. It is not easy. Anxiety can come flooding in, despite the reassurances provided by professionals and the efforts of healthcare staff and other front-line workers. There are ways to manage this anxiety: staying informed but limiting media consumption, watching our diet and exercise patterns, trying to get some sleep and reaching out to others, using technology if necessary.

By now, we have all seen communities rise to the occasion over the past two years of Covid-19: setting up groups on-line, supporting the isolated and sharing our worries and strengths with each other. We are fortunate that most (although not all) cases of Covid-19 are now self-limiting, if unpleasant. We know that the situation is improving, if still far from stable. There is real hope this month—we can almost taste it.

Over this period, we have seen many Irish politicians step up to the mark, change their work practices and take full responsibility for our response to the pandemic. That is exactly what we need: adults in the room, along with our superb public health officials and impressive bunch of scientists. Many public figures have stood up straight and said their piece, even if others have yet to learn this skill. They will.

So, while more people will get the virus, even at this late stage, and, sadly, more will die, healthcare staff continue to perform quiet miracles in their places of work, supported by other front-line workers across society. I see this happen every day. I never cease to be astonished by it. This is an extraordinary time.

We know that all health systems are imperfect. Even prior to Covid-19, virtually every country in the world needed more doctors, nurses, allied health professionals, inpatient beds, primary care, mental health services, social supports and community facilities. These problems will remain long after Covid-19 has passed.

If the pandemic has shown us anything, however, it is that, despite these issues, healthcare staff have no shortage of spirit, no lack of imagination and no deficit of commitment. I am humbled by what I see, more thankful than I can say, and deeply impressed at the positive changes in healthcare workplaces over the past two years. Revolution was needed. Revolution came.

There are, of course, costs and downsides to these changes. Emergency care for Covid-19 elbowed out other needs and services over the past two years. While it is difficult to measure the impact of a delayed hip operation or deferred cataract surgery, it is substantial.[58] As the pandemic hopefully subsides, it is essential that we recognise these knock-on effects on the health system and rebalance our priorities so that the world regains some of its equilibrium.

Even so, there is no doubt that medical workplaces have changed for the foreseeable future and possibly forever.

We have seen not only increased use of technology and greater flexibility but also the system's ability to respond to a crisis—something that few thought possible prior to the pandemic. The health system surprised itself. Who knew this could happen?

There is a broader lesson here, as many other workplaces changed too.[59] All across the world, workers camped out in spare rooms, plonked laptops on kitchen tables and upgraded their WiFi. This amounted to a fascinating, if inadvertent, experiment in changing work practices very quickly at a uniquely complicated time in many people's lives.[60]

The outcomes of this mass experiment were by no means guaranteed, not least because working from home presents a challenge to both 'work' and 'home'. Usually, home is where we go to escape from work. So, if we work at home, boundaries become more important than ever. There was a real possibility that these changes would be a general disaster, and everyone would scurry back to their physical workplace at the first opportunity, happy to leave home behind.

In the event, the experiment in home working had a positive outcome for many people. For a significant proportion of workers, the shift towards home changed how they view their work and how they understand balance in their lives. For others, the limits of home working were soon apparent, as home duties, especially childcare, were simply added in on top of work and quickly became unmanageable. For some, chaos ensued.

One good technique to manage the situation was to 'commute' to work at home. In other words, at 9 a.m. some home workers put on their coats, went outside, walked around the block for ten minutes and then arrived back home to 'work'. They did likewise at 5 p.m. in order to 'come home from work'. This helped to reset minds and bodies, even if the working day was still interrupted by children, deliveries, cooking, laundry and a certain amount of home life. The symbolism of commuting helps and is especially useful for letting go of work at 5 p.m. We need limits.

The bigger issue that arose concerned human connection. The mass experiment in home working demonstrated beyond doubt that many people go to their workplaces not to work (it turns out that much of that can be done from home) but in order to chat with colleagues, loiter at the water-cooler, gather in the carpark and exchange news after meetings.[61] These activities are essential for organic team-building, generating new ideas and optimising group performance. We need each other. It is difficult to gossip at a meeting on-line.

Overall, perhaps, the greatest insight from these changes is that working from home proved more possible than many people might have imagined. The other insight is that working from home is not simple. It is important to separate home work from 'work' work as much as feasible, and to connect informally with colleagues. As more people move back into physical workplaces after the pandemic, opportunities for social and semi-social activities should be prioritised, rather than focusing exclusively on core work. We need to connect with colleagues just as much as we need to work with them, if not more so. Chatting keeps us together.

In the end, it turns out that work is as much about emotion, values and networks as it is about work. This fact is even more apparent among a younger generation who commonly struggle with a toxic combination of zero-hour contracts, job insecurity, accommodation problems and increasingly precarious financial situations.[62] This is a substantial challenge for society and the future of work.

Traditionally, the first half of life is concerned with tasks such as forming relationships, shaping a career, establishing a home and consolidating a sense of self. All of these activities are more challenging today owing to issues as diverse as altered patterns of wealth transfer between generations and unhelpful developments in property markets. Add in the socially distorting effects of a pandemic and the current era becomes an especially difficult time to be young.

President Michael D. Higgins addressed this issue in 2019, before the pandemic, when he spoke at the Congress of the European Federation of Public Service Unions:

I am minded to re-visit the related philosophical concept of 'The Dignity of Labour', much advocated by Gandhi, in which all types of jobs are respected equally, no occupation is considered superior, and none of the jobs should be discriminated on any basis; is this not the ethic of work in the public service for the public good?

I believe a corollary of this concept is that a return to the fundamentals of decent, secure jobs would be a widespread increase in job satisfaction, a better sense of accomplishment, and improvements in quality of life across nations. A vision in which these concepts become more embedded in the citizenry, and, in particular, employers, is perhaps provocative, even radical, as it attempts to upturn the commonly held assertion that money and wealth accumulation is the primary motivation behind humans' desire to work.[63]

President Higgins is right. Work is about a great deal more than 'money and wealth accumulation', as Covid-19 demonstrated.

The emergency phase of the pandemic clearly underlined 'the dignity of labour' and the importance of work as part of the social contract, an essential element in our connectedness. This applies not only to front-line workers but also to everyone whose work contributes to the running of their family, their community and our societies more broadly. We are inter-related beings in ways that we might not have imagined prior to Covid-19. We need each other more profoundly than we ever knew.

Work is also, for many people, part of our identities and a key component of how we view our lives. Although we should not overburden work with meaning or symbolism, work inevitably matters to us as individuals, be that work inside the home, outside the home or—increasingly, during the pandemic—a mixture of both.

Work also reflects our moods and various phases of our lives. Wilde struggled with work after the Travers case in

1864. While he continued to see large numbers of patients, he was less courteous and gracious with them.[64] This was perhaps understandable to a degree, but was also regrettable, and marked a deterioration in standards for Wilde. Further difficulty followed when his 9-year-old daughter Isola died, most likely of an infection, in 1867. This was one of the great tragedies of Wilde's life. He was not the same after it.

During this period, following the trial, Wilde spent lengthy periods away from Dublin, albeit working busily. In 1867 he published one of his finest books, *Lough Corrib, its Shores and Islands: with Notices of Lough Mask*.[65] This earned him the Cunningham Gold Medal of the Royal Irish Academy. In the volume, he clearly luxuriates in the heritage and countryside of the west of Ireland which was so dear to him. Here, he describes the ruins of a Franciscan Friary in Claregalway:

> When the sun breaks forth after a passing shower, brightening up a side of this tower, and throwing out the gorgeous colours of golden lichen clothing its grey time-beaten stones, and contrasting with the brilliant green of the pellitory and umbelliferous plants that cluster on its string courses, and around its windows and corbied parapet, a more glorious effect, and at the same time a more beauteous harmony of colour and form, can scarcely be imagined.[66]

This is Wilde letting his powers of description run riot, a desperate desire for escape evident in his quasi-mystical engagement with the Irish countryside. He details his travels with a keen eye not only for nature but also for man's impact on the surroundings—and the tension between the two:

> A cold, wet day—and such is not uncommon in this district—with the mist drifting along the mountains, renders the drive, from Ballinahinch to the village of Oughterard, not over-pleasant to the tourist who occupies the windy side of an outside car, of either long or short dimensions. As we approach Oughterard through other properties, the *débris* of mining operations show that capital, energy, and enterprise, are still required for a line of country, along whose magnificent road we well remember, in our early fishing days, to have seen a goodly sprinkling of snug cottages, potato fields, and cabbage gardens,—where now the bog has again grown up, and the purple heather, and yellow asphodel, and other wild flowers of nature, are hourly turning back to its original state what the spade and the strong arm had rendered subservient to the service of man.[67]

Seized by Wilde's descriptions and story, I go to see his beloved home at Moytura, near the village of Cong in County Mayo. Wilde had taken to spending an increasing amount of time here, even prior to the 1864 trial.[68] Today, I can see why; it is a beautiful spot: calm, leafy, lakeside. Poet Padraic Colum set his 1963 play *Moytura: A Play for Dancers* here, featuring Wilde and dedicated to Wilde's biographer, T.G. Wilson.[69]

Moytura House is privately owned, so I cannot access the grounds. Instead, I visit Cong village and go to the Catholic graveyard in the village centre. The burial-ground is just opposite the ruins of the old Church of Ireland church. I see a memorial plaque on the boundary wall:

> To the memory of
> Mary Burke
> Who died at Moytura May 1870
> Aged 85
> She was for 50 years
> The faithful servant and
> Attached friend of the family of
> Sir William R. Wilde,
> By whom this tablet
> Has been erected
> In grateful recollection.
> R.I.P.

Later in February, I travel beyond Cong and leave Ireland for the first time in two years. I spend a glorious, snowy week in Iceland: Reykjavik, geysers, hot springs. There is ice everywhere. The temperature is subzero. I experience two days of red weather warnings. The wind is majestic and terrifying.

The entire experience in Iceland is elemental and untutored. I missed this during Covid-19: the thrill of the foreign.

Travel is different during the pandemic.[70] It is more negotiated and uncertain, but it is glorious to be reminded that the world is big—bigger than me, bigger than Ireland, bigger than Covid-19.

Back home in central Dublin, life re-emerges. Late one evening, after dusk, I stand outside my house with a cup of tea, thinking about things.

Suddenly, I hear scuffling from a nearby tree. I discern the outline of a large bird landing on a branch, arranging its wings. I take a closer look. Slowly, the bird turns its head to reveal the characteristic shape of an owl's face. I have never seen an owl in the wild before. The moment is magical, like something in a dream, part of a fairy tale, or a fragment of some different life, imagined.

I am transfixed. It does not occur to me to take a photo with my phone. The experience is too immediate, too real, too precious.

The owl looks at me, blinks, glances around, spreads its wings and disappears over the rooftops, into the dark. The incident lasts no more than three minutes, but it transforms my night, my week, my year, my life.

I saw an owl.

5. SPRING 2022: RESOLUTION

'Healing is a matter of time, but it is sometimes also a matter of opportunity.'

–Hippocrates

*T*his chapter takes us from March to May 2022 and looks to the future, examining what we might learn from the Covid-19 pandemic. The most likely outcome is that, as a society, we will learn virtually nothing. From a historical perspective, individuals remember but societies forget. That said, if any lessons do emerge from the past few years, five key points are likely to rank among them. The first is that infection is eternal and will rise again—and this will probably happen sooner rather than later if we continue to dangerously unbalance our planet. The second point is that numbers, statistics and science matter deeply, especially when our worlds are turned upside down by an event like Covid-19. We know this now more than ever. The third lesson is that, despite the enormous value of numbers and statistics, stories matter too, both to illustrate the importance of research findings and for more profound, human reasons: in a crisis, we are hungry for narrative and meaning. We need the world to make sense (even if it doesn't). The fourth lesson is that our way of life is more fragile than many people in rich countries previously realised, but we are also stronger than we thought. The pandemic demonstrated our enormous resilience in the face of terrible suffering. Finally, escape is vital: losing ourselves in favourite activities or leaving our worlds behind us when we travel—just as William Wilde did with his lifelong obsessions with busyness, statistics and stories, and his love of touring. Also in this chapter, I loiter in Merrion Square, climb two mountains and see a squirrel doing something that I did not know squirrels could do.

MARCH 2022

Spring arrives in March. For Emerson, this month is as unsettled as the affairs of life: 'Our life is March weather, savage and serene in one hour'. March brings the festival of Saint Patrick, who banished snakes from Ireland in the fifth century and whose walking-stick took root as a tree. For some, the transitions of March are less dramatic, but they are no less profound. Lucy Maud Montgomery writes that 'March came in that winter like the meekest and mildest of lambs, bringing days that were crisp and golden and tingling, each followed by a frosty pink twilight which gradually lost itself in an elfland of moonshine'. That is my March: gentle frost, golden days and tingling joys of moonlight.

We emerge, gingerly. Restrictions lightened, I make a trip to the Heritage Centre of the Royal College of Physicians of Ireland (RCPI) at 6 Kildare Street in Dublin.[1] The RCPI Heritage Centre preserves, protects and promotes the College's collections relating to the history of medicine and medical education in Ireland. These collections include thousands of books, pamphlets, photographs, artworks, medical instruments and other unique items collected since the College's foundation in 1654. That's a long time.

The RCPI Heritage Centre is one of Ireland's hidden gems, a treasure trove of historical texts, antique medical equipment and—wait for it—Napoleon's toothbrush.[i] The Centre includes the beautiful, book-lined 'Dun's Library' that has been part of the College since 1713, when Sir Patrick Dun (1642–1713), an eminent physician and former RCPI president, bequeathed his personal library to create this astonishing collection. Since 2020 I have been 'Dun's Librarian' and I continually come across new wonders in the storerooms. They are infinite.

Today, in the glorious quiet of the Heritage Centre reading room, I contemplate a letter from Sir William Wilde to George Petrie (1790–1866), an Irish painter, musician, antiquarian and archaeologist who, like Wilde, was involved with the collections of the Royal Irish Academy (on nearby Dawson Street). Wilde wrote this letter to Petrie on 14 December 1858, in his home on Merrion Square. The short note in front of me provides a fascinating insight into the

i   I'm not joking.

scope of Wilde's interests, as he enthuses breathlessly about 'sword handles' that he came across in Scandinavia during one of his many forays abroad:

My dear Petrie,

The accompanying is a transcript of memoranda I made respecting sword handles when in Scandinavia. Pray remember that they are very rough, the mere dictation from my notes upon my return […] I covet a drawing of your sword handle because it is *Irish* and because it is *yours* […] I long to tell you of the marvels I saw in Scandinavia but on the one hand, time presses hard upon one these short dark days, and on the other hand I fear to intrude or press upon you […]

Yours, & c.,

W.R. Wilde[2]

Wilde had an extraordinary mind, always hungry for facts, figures, details and understanding.[3] This brief letter is just one glimpse into his kaleidoscopic inner world, a random sample from the constant churn of communications, thoughts and activities that filled his multi-faceted, multi-layered, multi-coloured life. Wilde saw 'marvels' not only in Scandinavia but everywhere he looked. His ability to marvel was, perhaps, the greatest marvel of all.

It is not difficult to see where his children got some of their brilliance. The RCPI Heritage Collection provides much insight into the great man's work: letters, books, images, and even prescriptions in Wilde's handwriting. Gazing at these today, it feels as if Wilde is sitting right here beside me in Kildare Street, probably wondering what I'm doing here.[ii]

The Heritage Centre collections are always growing. Just as the College collected material relating to Wilde and others over past centuries, we recently sought to capture the experiences of people working in healthcare during Covid-19.[4] We encouraged healthcare workers to share their experiences in written, audio or video format, submitting letters, diaries, video diaries or other material. We also put out a call for visual material or other items that relate to Covid-19, such as photographs, drawings, newspaper cuttings, poetry or creative work. Anything, really, to capture the moment.

This contemporaneous record continues to grow and will hopefully help future historians to understand this terrible, extraordinary pandemic. Already, in early 2022, as the emergency subsides in certain countries, people are trying to figure out what, if anything, we have learned from our experiences. Are the lessons of Covid-19 apparent? Will they ever be? Have we learned anything? Do we ever learn anything?

While it is too early to reach firm conclusions, we must consider the possibility that societies will learn virtually nothing from Covid-19.[5] Despite the upheaval and suffering, it remains possible that no lessons will emerge, or, if they do, we will not learn them—or, if we do, we will forget them. In broad terms, the history of previous pandemics suggests that this is a likely outcome and that

ii   I'm wondering, too.

we will quickly go back to behaving how we did prior to Covid-19.[6] By this reasoning, any 'lessons' that 'society' might 'learn' in the short term will soon be forgotten. Virtually everything in society will revert to how it was before the pandemic.

The problem is not so much that the pandemic didn't have an impact—it clearly did—but that we, as societies, tend not to 'learn' lessons. As individuals we learn lots, but as groups virtually nothing. During Covid-19 we learned from private, personal tragedies, not public ones.[7] While the pandemic provided the backdrop to everything in our lives, specific losses were rooted in individual circumstances.

History is clear: group learning simply does not occur in these situations, even after pandemics. Or, if it does happen in the short term, it does not last. As individuals, we remember. As societies, we forget—and we forget with unnerving speed.

That said, it is still useful to think about the aftermath of Covid-19 at the level of society and to see whether detailed accounts of responses to the pandemic offer any insights, especially for countries still struggling with the virus. There are now many such accounts of various aspects of Covid-19.[8] More appear almost daily.[iii] It is likely that Covid-19 will continue to be debated and explored for many decades, if not centuries, to come, as is the case with the 1918 influenza pandemic.[9]

Many reflections over the past two years focus on broad-sweep 'lessons' that we probably should have learned prior

iii   I appreciate that I am contributing to this deluge of reflection.

to Covid-19 but which were (arguably) highlighted by the pandemic. Journalist Fareed Zakaria outlines *Ten Lessons for a Post-Pandemic World*, including that humans are social animals, globalisation has not died and quality of government matters more than quantity.[10] Economist Rebecca Henderson writes about *Reimagining Capitalism in a World on Fire*, arguing that Covid-19 pushed this topic to centre stage.[11] Former UK Prime Minister Gordon Brown proposes *Seven Ways to Change the World*, including focusing on global health, growth, the environment, education, sustainable development, inequality and nuclear disarmament.[12] Former Governor of the Bank of England Mark Carney writes about social and economic values in *Value(s): Building a Better World for All*, arguing in favour of a life of purpose, morality and humility.[13]

Many of these points might reasonably have been made prior to the pandemic, but Covid-19 appears to have given them added immediacy. These things always mattered, but it feels like they matter more now—and maybe they do.

Looking more specifically at the past two years, Scott Galloway, an author and professor of marketing, argues that shocks like pandemics and wars are painful but are often followed by especially productive periods in human history.[14] This might or might not prove to be the case with Covid-19.

Another volume, *Rethink: Leading Voices on Life After Crisis and How We Can Make a Better World*, edited by Amol Rajan, presents diverse thoughts from such figures as Pope Francis, Brian Eno and Samantha Power on a broad range of topics that (they argue) need to be rethought after the emergency is over.[15] These issues range from poverty to global governance, from the body to digital power. Again, many of these insights are valid and valuable, even if most clearly pre-date the pandemic. Only time will tell how much rethinking actually happens as a direct result of Covid-19—very little, I suspect. Or, if change occurs, it will be less conscious, more organic and not in the directions anticipated. History tends to be non-linear, to say the least.

In the end, Covid-19 changed much in our societies, but not everything. The pandemic was first and foremost a public health emergency rather than an existential crisis. While its philosophical implications should not be ignored, and can be explored in time, it is important not to overburden the coming years with exaggerated expectations of revelation, revolution and reform. Yes, we need to build back better, but the first step is starting to build back at all.

With all this reflection, theorising and opportunistic pushing of old agendas, it is important to remain focused on the facts about Covid-19 and not get distracted from what the outbreak really was: an enormous public health problem; a scaring personal tragedy for the ill and bereaved; a financial catastrophe for others, especially those who lost their jobs; and a salutary reminder about the fragility of our way of life, brought into shattering focus by a tiny virus that uses invisibility as a weapon.[16]

Covid-19 was also an apparent vindication for the prophets of doom who routinely predict that gross misfortune is about to befall the world. The naysayers are usually wrong, but on random occasions they are correct. While this was one of those occasions, that does not mean that the pessimists had any basis for their predictions.

Against this background, it is little surprise that the pandemic has prompted a great deal of expansive speculation and far-fetched theorising. Does Covid-19 signal the end of globalisation as we know it? Is the planet striking back against our vicious environmental vandalism? Does Covid-19 present an existential threat to the very idea of what it means to be human?

These questions are valid and relevant to varying degrees, and there is little doubt that there is a philosophical and spiritual side to any experience of this nature.[17] We certainly need to slow down and contemplate what just happened.[iv]

But if this period of reflection highlights any lessons—and, as mentioned, it might not—it is likely that these lessons will be smaller and simpler but more powerful than is commonly imagined. Rather than entering the arenas of complex philosophical or existential exploration, then, let's start with the first lesson, which is also the simplest and the one that is most often overlooked, even today: infection is eternal. We ignore this at our peril.

During his lifetime, William Wilde learned only too much about the power of infection from his clinical career as a doctor, his work on the census and his personal life, especially the loss of his daughter Isola to meningitis in 1867. In the census reports, Wilde devoted particular attention to

iv   Thus, this.

accounts of infections and plagues in the *Annals of the Four Masters*, which he adored. At one point Wilde commissioned a stone cross commemorating the Masters, which still resides in the Four Masters Park in Phibsborough, Dublin.[18] It is well worth a visit.

In his 'Table of Cosmical Phenomena, Epizootics, Famines, and Pestilences in Ireland' in the 1851 census report, Wilde quotes the Four Masters linking God with a deadly 'pestilence' in 1044:

> Cluain-mic-Nois was plundered by the Conmhaicni; and God and Ciaran wreaked great vengeance upon them for it, i.e., an unknown plague [*Tamh anaithinadh*] was sent among them, so that the Booleys [dairies or summer houses] were left waste with their cattle, after the death of all the [shepherd] people.[19]

Another 'horrid unknown disease' is recounted in the *Annals of Clonmacnois* in the same year, attributed—again—to God:

> For which outrages committed upon the clergy of St Queran, God horribly plagued them with a horrid unknown disease, that they died so fast of that infection that their towns, houses [...] were altogether waste without men or cattle.[20]

In 1240 St Maula was involved in another puzzling outbreak, which Wilde describes with a quote from *Hanmer's Chronicle*:

There was a great plague in that towne [Kilkenny], and such as died thereof, being bound with wythes [ropes or cords] upon the beere [coffin], were buried in St Maulas (Mother to St Kennis) churchyard; after that the infection ceased; women and maids went thither to dance, and instead of handkerchiefs and napkins to keepe them together in their round, it is said they took those wythes to serve their purpose. It is generally received (take it, gentle reader, as cheape as you find it) that Maula was angry for profaning her churchyard, and with the wythes infected the dancers, so that shortly after, in Kilkenny, there died of the sickness man, woman, and child.[21]

Wilde cautions that 'from the foregoing extract it is difficult to pronounce as to whether this epidemic was the true Bubonic Plague, or an outbreak of the Dancing Mania, then prevalent in Europe'. The *Report of Cork Street Hospital* is clearer about the causes of a different outbreak in Dublin in the early 1800s:

A gradual increase of fever in Dublin during the years 1812, '13, and '14 is shown by the reports of Cork Street Fever Hospital; and, says Dr O'Brien, 'We behold its quantity annually multiplied, and its ravages extended, as those causes which are universally allowed to be the great promoters of infection among the poor still exist with augmented energy; these are want, filth, crowded apartments, idleness, dejection, intoxication'.[22]

There is remarkable similarity between these factors fuelling infection in the early 1800s and the forces driving Covid-19 two centuries later. Poverty and inequality are still chief among these, as arguments and discussions about pandemics reverberate consistently through the ages.[23] Proposed solutions are similar, too. Here is Wilde again, quoting advice from the 1800s that might equally apply in the context of Covid-19:

> Houses of recovery succeed only partially in the prevention of infection, by curing infected persons, contracting the sphere of contagion, and lessening the mortality; but [an] efficient system of police is absolutely necessary to give an effectual and permanent check to its progress. [The present system of Metropolitan Police was not introduced until 1838, and the first Sanitary Association was established in 1848.]
>
> The object of such a system would be to encourage cleanliness (the great antidote to contagion) among the poor, to clear the wretched receptacles in which they dwell of their accumulated filth, to discourage residence in cellars, and to excite industry, the parent of cleanliness and sobriety; to provide work for the unemployed ...[24]

Bill Gates, in *How to Prevent the Next Pandemic*, recommends not only better preparedness for pandemics after Covid-19 but also closing the health gap between the rich and the poor, just as Wilde and others recognised almost two centuries earlier.[25] Infection is intrinsically social and is therefore partly preventable through social means: better housing, better sanitation, better healthcare, and equal opportunities for work and social progress.[26] Vaccines are an enormous advance, but they need to be accompanied by public health and social reform if they are to achieve their full potential.

This should not have come as a surprise with Covid-19, even based on recent history. Social conditions have always mattered deeply and continue to matter today. Drug-resistant infections killed almost 1.3 million people globally in 2019, just prior to the pandemic, with the highest toll in sub-Saharan Africa.[27] Even within rich countries, economic disparities and social roles matter a lot. In *Preventable: How a Pandemic Changed the World and How to Stop the Next One*, Devi Sridhar, Professor and Chair of Global Public Health at the University of Edinburgh, points to three risk factors for death from Covid-19: having a deprived background; coming from a racial or ethnic minority group; and having an occupation such as security guard, cleaner, taxi driver, healthcare or social care worker.[28] Infection is eternal, but its impact is very social.

So, how did Ireland fare during Covid-19? Despite the undeniable negative impact, the trauma and the losses, did we manage the pandemic well compared to other countries? Or were there obvious failings that we might have avoided?

These are difficult questions that were continually (and rightly) posed in the white heat of the pandemic. During the longest and most difficult periods, a great deal of attention focused on the actions of the government and its public health advisors. When there was bad news, we tended to blame the communication process between the government and the National Public Health Emergency Team (NPHET) or seek evidence that the government was more responsible for the situation than it actually was.[29]

Commentators demanded 'clarity' when clarity was clearly impossible. Industry leaders asked for 'certainty' in a uniquely uncertain world. When they got neither, anger erupted. NPHET and the government were blamed.

The atmosphere was febrile, but while such criticism might have been appropriate to a certain extent, there was a good deal of displacement going on. In other words, much of the frustration that was directed against NPHET and the government would have been more accurately aimed at the virus itself.

Blaming a virus does not, however, fulfil the psychological need to hold a person responsible, so we shifted our anger to politicians, the government, NPHET or the media. Unsatisfying as it might be, though, it was the virus that we should have blamed much more than we did. These other actors played far lesser roles.

The same could be said about the social and economic impact of Covid-19. It was primarily the pandemic that was unfair, not NPHET or the government. Like most infections, Covid-19 presents the greatest risk to older adults and people with pre-existing illnesses. This intrinsic unfairness echoed through all aspects of the pandemic but was mostly attributable to the biology of the virus rather than actions taken or not taken by NPHET or our politicians.

Globally, most of those who died of Covid-19 died of a combination of infection, poverty and injustice. In Ireland and elsewhere, sectors of the economy that did not rely on groups and gatherings were considerably less risky than those that did, such as hospitality, sports and live entertainment. This was desperately unfair on people who work in these sectors, but the unfairness was biological, not political.

As a medical doctor, I was privileged to have a job and to be vaccinated early in the vaccination programme. Not everyone was so lucky. The virus, like most of nature, was—and is—grotesquely unfair. It is important that government policies do not amplify this injustice, but the intrinsic, baseline unfairness lies with the pandemic itself, not the politicians or public health officials who try to manage it.

In fact, it is now clear that, despite the challenges, hesitations and various complexities, Ireland's management of the pandemic compares well to other countries.[30] Infection might be eternal but responses vary. While the suffering and losses were enormous, Ireland still did better than most other places around the world, at least in terms of deaths.

A systematic analysis in *The Lancet* medical journal reports that the Covid-19 mortality rate was 120.3 excess deaths per 100,000 of the population globally.[31] Rates varied a great deal across different countries, with the highest rate reported in Bolivia (734.9). Ireland's rate was notably low, at 12.5 excess deaths per 100,000 owing to Covid-19. The

UK rate was far higher, at 126.8. While various factors (such as population structure) influence these figures, other measures of outcomes generally confirm that the impact of Covid-19 in Ireland was well below European and global averages.[32] This is good news.

While there were clearly many tragedies, and the political response was occasionally less than polished, Ireland did not do too badly as a country, at least in the emergency period. As a result, today, at the end of March 2022, our Covid-19 restrictions are the second lightest in the world.[33] This is a real achievement, attributable to both the actions of the Irish people during lockdown after lockdown and the work of politicians and public health officials who held their nerve at critical moments. This was not easy for anyone, and everyone played a part. Vaccination was a life-saver.

The picture in the longer term is less predictable. While it is hoped that vaccines reduce the risk of long Covid, it is not yet clear whether the Irish health system has learned systematic lessons from the pandemic or whether we are prepared for further waves.[34] What is evident, however, from this pandemic and from previous ones is that there will be more outbreaks of Covid-19 or something similar in the future. Infection is eternal. It goes away, but it comes back. We need to be more ready.

To compound matters, it is now clear that most of humanity's problems are linked with each other in profound and powerful ways. Climate change is probably the greatest threat we face.[35] As such, it is inevitably linked with the risk of future pandemics. Writing in *The Guardian*, Jonathan Watts joins the dots in no uncertain terms:

> The interconnectedness of the world's crises is increasingly apparent. Epidemiologists and conservationists have warned that outbreaks of coronavirus-like diseases are more likely in the future as a result of deforestation, global heating and humankind's treatment of nature [...] Despite new vaccines, a new US president, a newfound respect for science and a new awareness of how rapidly change can come, it remains to be seen whether this crisis will lead to transformation—or more tinkering around the edges.[36]

APRIL 2022

April is mid-spring. For Shakespeare, this month puts 'a spirit of youth in everything'. It opens with April Fool's Day, when 'we remember what we are the other 364 days of the year', according to Mark Twain. We are always fools in one way or another—and even greater fools to forget this for so much of the year. But April is more than a salutary reminder of folly. Christopher Columbus, in his Journal of First Voyage to America, *wrote about 'air soft as that of Seville in April, and so fragrant that it was delicious to breathe it'. April is a time of promise, change, discovery. For Thoreau, April baptises the season: 'Spring. March fans it, April christens it, and May puts on its jacket and trousers.'*

Hope continues to grow in Ireland, even as this terrible pandemic rages mercilessly in certain parts of the world and gradually subsides in others. If the first lesson of Covid-19 is that infection is eternal, this realisation needs to be weighed against the resilience, hope and survival that have been so apparent over the past two years. It was always thus, even during the Spanish 'flu, which caused the deaths of over 50 million people around the world, including more than 20,000 in Ireland, over a century ago.[37] Hope survived then, too.

As a psychiatrist, I have an abiding interest in Sigmund Freud. In January 1920 Freud's daughter, Sophie, fell victim to the 'flu in Hamburg. Two days after her death, Freud wrote that 'the undisguised brutality of our time is weighing heavily upon us'.[38] Just like Covid-19, the Spanish 'flu saw a great many people struggle with loss of life, loss of livelihood and loss of hope. Nevertheless, like today, many people found ways to abide, adapt and survive, even in the face of unthinkable loss.

Both then and now, the suffering was very real, but so is the tenacity of the human spirit. Freud saw cause for hope in logical thought and considered action. 'The benefits of order are incontestable', he later wrote.[39] Also, presciently: 'We are not surprised by the idea of setting up the use of soap as an actual yardstick of civilisation'. Never is this truer than during an outbreak like the Spanish 'flu or Covid-19 today.

As with the 1918 'flu, 'the undisguised brutality of our time' has dominated our recent past but is hopefully diminishing now, hastened by vaccination, public health measures, economic interventions and deep compassion for all who suffer. As Freud pointed out, 'the healing power of love … is not to be despised'.[40] We are always better together.

One of the key features of the current pandemic has been the centrality of numbers, statistics and science in our understanding of the virus and our public discourse about how to respond. This is, perhaps, the second key lesson from the Covid-19 pandemic (if there are any lessons): that numbers matter, statistics matter and science matters deeply, now more than ever.

Pandemics and diseases have a unique ability to change how we see the world. For Wilde, scientifically informed practice was the key to understanding and alleviating suffering from all kinds of ill health and misfortune.[41] Hence Wilde's clinical work, his love of statistics and his devotion to the census reports, especially their analysis of infectious diseases through the ages.

Wilde was especially interested in patterns of disease transmission and how to interrupt the spread of infection. He quotes *Graves' Report upon Fever in Galway and the West of Ireland* from 1822, when there was a 'partial famine' owing to 'general failure of the potato crop' and 'the spring and summer fisheries proved unproductive'. The 'increase of fever, and the mortality consequent thereon, began to attract attention in the month of May', especially around Galway:

During the months of June, July, and August, all parts of the town and adjacent country, with the exception of Claddagh village, had become affected; and much alarm was excited, as well by the rapid diffusion of the disease among the poor as by its spreading to the upper classes of society, in which the proportion of deaths was much greater, amounting to nearly one-third of those attacked. The disease increased towards the end of Autumn.

Ropes were stretched across the streets to prevent the passage of cars or carriages, which might by their noise disturb the sick. The terror of infection was so great that it was not unusual for persons to guard their mouths with handkerchiefs while passing those houses in which a case of fever was known to exist. The shops of such as had any member of their family unwell were almost deserted. Many persons living in the country were afraid to purchase clothes or other articles in the town.[42]

This anxiety and fear, and the measures taken to avoid infection, are only too familiar from the past two years of Covid-19. We also recognise Wilde's desire to understand how much infection is present, why it spreads and what the risks are. With Covid-19, our efforts to comprehend these things focused largely on numbers, as the news reported daily statistics about cases, hospitalisations and deaths. Sometimes it felt as if the numbers would never end.

Against this background it was easy to become obsessed, checking data from distant countries around the world (no matter how misleading comparisons with Ireland were), following obscure statistics over time (even though data collection varied a great deal, making trends difficult to interpret), or—all too often—searching for the most negative and depressing statistics we could find (even though we knew we should not). All told, many people clung to statistics for dear life, interpreting day-to-day fluctuations as disasters (if they were negative) or cause for celebration (if positive). It was exhausting.

In truth, numbers shifted quite slowly, no matter how much our worried minds tried to interpret every twitch in the statistics. Deep down, most people knew this, but numbers offer a kind of safety. The daily statistics at media briefings suggested that, while the pandemic might feel infinite and uncontrolled, it could, at the very least, be measured. And that was enough to help many of us through the bad times. While we might not have figured out how to stop it yet, at least someone knew the size and shape of the problem. There was real comfort in that.

In addition to this psychological and emotional value, of course, statistics really did help to describe, understand and address Covid-19. For me, a 2021 book by David Spiegelhalter and Anthony Masters, *Covid by Numbers: Making Sense of the Pandemic with Data*, helped me navigate the kaleidoscopic world of Covid-19 statistics with an appreciation of both the limits and the value of numbers.[43] Not everything can be counted, but much can.

In their book, Spiegelhalter and Masters provide a careful, no-nonsense guide to all kinds of statistics about the virus, including diagnoses, cases, interventions, reactions and vaccines. As they comment in *The Observer*, numbers are a key part of the impact of Covid-19 on our lives:

Individual experiences and suffering are, of course, at the heart of the pandemic. But one way to understand what has happened is through putting those experiences together— and statistics are those personal stories writ large. And this pandemic has brought unprecedented demand to explain all the numbers that have been flying around [...]

Unfortunately, this pandemic has been rife with false claims and misinformation, particularly about vaccines. One approach for dealing with this, supported by empirical evidence, is the idea of 'inoculation'—pre-empting misinformation and telling people about the incorrect interpretation before they catch it in the wild.[44]

Spiegelhalter and Masters are particularly useful on the subject of vaccination. They write that the roll-out of vaccines has been an incredible success story, to the point that it is terrifying to imagine what would have happened without them. As the *New Scientist* confirms, ending this pandemic depends on vaccination rates, evolution of the virus, advances in treatment and preventing infection through public health measures such as social distancing and ventilation.[45] Vaccines are central to much of this.

But while I am convinced by overwhelming scientific evidence in favour of vaccines, not everyone shares my view of the world. Some people are more affected by personal stories and metaphors than by numbers and charts. I love numbers to the extent that I am emotionally moved by statistics, profoundly affected by well-presented graphs and motivated to action by time-series data. At one point I studied epidemiology with an enthusiasm that was frankly disturbing.[v] This experience hugely enhanced my respect for statistics. I just love numbers.

Despite this, I appreciate that individual stories and metaphors have greater impact than statistics for many people. In terms of metaphors, comparing the Covid-19 vaccine to a seat-belt in a car seemed especially accurate and compelling to me.[46] While the jab does not offer 100 per cent protection, it greatly diminishes risk, reduces harm and can save your life—just like a seat-belt.

Engaging with people who are vaccine-hesitant will prove crucial over the coming years to maintain progress against the virus.[47] Dialogue is vital, and listening is the most important part of dialogue. Some people declined vaccines in order to make a political point, rather than evaluating evidence about the risks of Covid-19 and the benefits of vaccination.[48] Some of us might find the science compelling, but science operates in the real world where people have complex histories, multiple concerns and different hopes for the future. Engagement, listening and acceptance help to increase trust, optimise exchange of views and chart a path forward for the benefit of all.

During Covid-19, statistics and science became part of this public dialogue in a way that was new for this generation. In Ireland we were fortunate to have a bunch of excellent scientists who engaged fully and openly in the

v   People worried about me.

public arena.[49] Not every country was so fortunate. We owe them a debt of gratitude.

So that, perhaps, is the second lesson that we might or might not learn from this pandemic: that numbers matter, statistics matter and science matters deeply, now more than ever. Of course, not all the numbers are in yet, and not all statistics are as clear as those about excess deaths and vaccination, both of which show Ireland doing comparatively well in international terms. Statistics in other areas are more difficult to interpret and might yet surprise us.

One of the most complex areas concerns my field of work, which is psychiatry, the branch of medicine devoted to treating mental illness. From this perspective, there is little doubt that the pandemic presented new and unfamiliar challenges to mental health services.[50] Nevertheless—as discussed in Chapter 4—I do not believe that Covid-19 triggered a pandemic of mental illness. There have been emotional challenges, diminished well-being, relapses into pre-existing conditions and lingering problems for some following Covid-19 infection. These are real challenges, but they do not constitute a pandemic of mental illness.[51] Detailed statistics about mental health tell a nuanced story of strengths and weaknesses, resilience and coping, suffering and support.

This less-dramatic picture is, perhaps, a surprise, given the turmoil, upheaval and losses that the virus inflicted on the world, but if the pandemic teaches us anything about prediction it is that we should be humble.[52] Efforts at projecting the course of this outbreak were, in one sense, essential, but they were also impossible (the virus presented constant surprises) and humbling (we do not control the world). Despite my weakness for a good statistic, even I admit that numbers are not the whole story, statistics can obsess us disproportionately and this virus repeatedly confounded all predictions. With this in mind, and as the situation improves here in Ireland, maybe we need to stop obsessing so much and start living more.[53] Finally, in April 2022, it is time.

This idea of limits to the value of statistics brings me to the third lesson that the pandemic might hold, if we are to learn any lessons from it (which we might not). The first lesson is that infection is eternal and will rise again—sooner rather than later, especially if we continue to dangerously unbalance our planet. The second lesson is that numbers, statistics and science matter deeply, particularly when we are scared. The third lesson is that, despite the enormous value of numbers, stories matter too—and not just to illustrate the importance of statistics but for more profound reasons as well. We are humans, not machines.

Wilde's story has always had a potent effect on me: his medical education, his clinical work, his immersion in the census and his colourful family. He died in 1876, many years before his son Oscar was convicted of gross indecency in 1895, served time in gaol and died of meningitis in 1900 (again, more infection, more tragedy). It is an extraordinary tale.

Today, the achievements of William Wilde are routinely overshadowed by Oscar's story and, when William is remembered, the tale of Mary Travers is commonly to the fore. This is attributable not only to Wilde's egregious behaviour towards Travers and the compelling nature of her story but also to the attraction of stories in general.[54] Narratives carry enormous weight. Stories, no matter how atypical, commonly outweigh other ways of understanding the world, such as facts, numbers and statistics—no matter how thrilling I might find a well-presented graph or how a statistic might make me swoon.[vi]

Today, I return to Wilde's family home at 1 Merrion Square to remember William's story and drink shots of toxic espresso beside Oscar's statue in the park. Adoring tourists take photographs of themselves in the leafy surrounds. Traffic thunders past. My pulse, thick with caffeine, quickens as the espressos take hold. I think about stories, memory and forgetting. Remembering keeps us alive; forgetting makes us human.

Even here, in Merrion Square, the story of William Wilde is not the only compelling narrative that was largely forgotten over time. In March 2021, a Dublin City Council committee voted to support the erection of a plaque to the memory of Violet Gibson, an Irish woman who shot Italian Fascist leader Benito Mussolini in 1926.[55] The plaque is located a few doors up from Wilde's house, at 12 Merrion Square, which was Gibson's childhood home.[56] Gibson's story is an intriguing one that merits close attention, as evidenced by recent interest in her life and deeds. It also fascinates me, as a psychiatrist.

---

vi   Again, I'm not joking. I sometimes feel a bit weak.

Gibson was born in 1876, the year that Wilde died. Her father, a lawyer and politician, became Baron Ashbourne in 1885. Her mother was a Christian Scientist. Gibson, like Oscar Wilde, enjoyed a relatively privileged upbringing here in Merrion Square.

Despite this advantage, she suffered from psychological problems for much of her life, often described as 'hysteria' but really quite unclear. These issues were compounded or fuelled by a series of bereavements, including the deaths of her fiancé, two brothers and a sister-in-law.

Gibson was plagued by infections and physical ill health: scarlet fever, pleurisy, Paget's disease and appendicitis. Treatments were less than precise, so she suffered from life-long complications of unsuccessful surgery.

Against this background, she increasingly turned to religions, both conventional and obscure, for meaning, solace and support. Notwithstanding these pursuits—or possibly because of them—her psychological problems persisted. Following the death of her brother, Victor, she spent time in a 'nursing home' in Kensington. She attacked her house-keeper's daughter with a knife, was certified insane and spent a period in Holloway Sanatorium in Surrey. Clearly, her problems had intensified.

In the mid-1920s, the combination of her life circumstances, the succession of bereavements and her chronic problems with physical and mental ill health became too much. In 1925 she attempted suicide in Rome, saying that she 'wanted to die for the glory of God'. Somehow she survived and went on, the following year, to etch her place in history.

In April 1926 Gibson brought a revolver with her to the Piazza del Campidoglio in Rome and shot at Benito Mussolini, just after he left an assembly of the International Congress of Surgeons. She fired twice, missing once and grazing the Fascist leader's nose with the other shot. If Mussolini had not turned his head just in time, she might well have killed him and changed the course of history. In the event, Mussolini was slightly injured and Gibson was taken away by the police.

Gibson said that she shot Mussolini 'to glorify God'. The Italian authorities eventually released her but returned her to the United Kingdom, where she was diagnosed with 'delusional insanity with paranoia'. She spent the remainder of her life in St Andrew's Psychiatric Hospital in Northampton.

Gibson's tragic, fascinating tale is recounted in full in an excellent historical biography by Frances Stonor Saunders, *The Woman Who Shot Mussolini*.[57] The Dublin City Council committee motion, from Councillor Mannix Flynn in December 2020, describes Gibson as 'a committed anti-fascist'.[58]

The 1920s, when Gibson was sent to St Andrew's, was a period in which large 'mental hospitals' were a feature of life in many parts of the world, including England and Ireland. Institutions and families collaborated to perpetuate admissions, often for decades. In 1952 Gibson's nephew, Edward, wrote to the doctor in Northampton to ask whether it was a statutory requirement for her to be visited twice a year. The doctor said that it was, so Edward said that he would fulfil the requirement but would only stay for 'a quarter of an hour or so'. Clearly, Gibson was very much alone, abandoned in the institution.

The decision to commemorate Gibson in Merrion Square is a welcome, interesting one. Her story is complex. From today's perspective, there is compelling evidence of psychological problems and even mental illness, but one must be careful about applying the diagnostic approaches of today to people in the past. The political dimensions of her case are enormous and were undoubtedly relevant to the outcome.

Today, I stand in Merrion Square and reflect on how some stories are mostly forgotten (William Wilde, Violet Gibson) but others are always remembered (Oscar Wilde). The fact that the decision to commemorate Gibson comes during a pandemic is significant. Narratives provide meaning at times of difficulty. In a crisis, we are hungry for stories.

The most iconic story of infection is probably Albert Camus's 1947 novel *La Peste* or *The Plague*.[59] This account of an outbreak in the town of 'Oran' is a classic tale that acquired mythic status during Covid-19, not least for its depiction of contrasting responses to quarantine and the hardships it imposes. Covid-19 is also producing a literature of its own, including poetry by Rita Ann Higgins and Chris Fitzpatrick that gives depth and context to the experience of the pandemic.[60]

All of this matters profoundly. Numbers matter. Stories matter. Language matters.[61] Meaning matters.[62]

Wilde understood this and, throughout his life, seamlessly integrated stories with statistics in his writing, his work on the census and his broader approach to other activities across many disciplines. More recently, President Michael D. Higgins emphasised 'pluralist scholarship' in a speech to the European Research Council at Iveagh House in October 2016:

> Indeed not through its physical properties alone can our universe or any of our lives together, or in lonely isolation, be understood. The humanities have something essential to contribute—alongside biology and neuroscience—to, for example, our comprehension of the nature of human consciousness or what it means to be human. It is through leaping the boundaries that divide discipline from discipline, science from the arts and humanities, and by marshalling the diverse influences from our intellectual heritage that we can best meet the complex challenges of the future, learn to live, and try to love.[63]

President Higgins returned to this topic at the University of Leipzig in July 2019, when he stressed 'that the required paradigm shift needs a space of epistemological freedom in our institutes of learning, by which I mean staff and students being allowed to think, university teachers given freedom to teach at least pluralistically, and fundamentally, free to critique a current orthodox capitalist system that is unregulated and unaccountable in its consequences for society and social policy'.[64] [vii] I am fortunate to enjoy this kind of freedom as a university teacher in Ireland, but not everyone is so lucky.

As I leave the storied Merrion Square today, I feel the impact of too many espressos subside in me. I reflect on the combination of numbers and stories that shape my view of the pandemic, my understanding of the world and my interest in Wilde. On the way home, I see a squirrel swim frantically across the canal and race across a busy road, narrowly escaping death. I never knew that squirrels could swim.

MAY 2022

May is a month of growth and, according to Sir Thomas Malory, 'the month when ... lovers, subject to the same force which reawakens the plants, feel their hearts open again, recall past trusts and past vows, and moments of tenderness, and yearn for a renewal of the magical awareness which is love'. For Shakespeare, May is 'full of spirit', although 'rough winds' can 'shake the darling buds of May'. Still, May is a time of beginnings, when summer lies ahead, full of promise. 'What potent blood hath modest May', wrote Emerson, who was born in May 1803. Potent blood indeed.

Potent blood or not, May 2022 brings continued optimism and hope, as the Covid-19 situation improves in Ireland, if

vii I have a weakness for President Higgins's speeches.

not elsewhere. May also brings me to the two final lessons that we might learn from Covid-19, although I'm still not convinced that we will learn anything as a society.

To summarise so far: the first lesson is that infection is eternal and will return. The second is that numbers, statistics and science matter deeply, especially in times of crisis. The third is that numbers alone are not enough: stories matter too, both to illustrate scientific truths and to move beyond figures, into the realm of narrative. We need to count, but we also need to dream.

The fourth lesson is that we are both more vulnerable and stronger than we think, and the fifth is that we all need to escape at times. We escape in mind by becoming absorbed in activities that occupy us and we escape in body by travelling outside our usual haunts to see the world. Climbing mountains is a good way to do both. First, though, before we escape to the hills, let's look at how Covid-19 highlighted our weaknesses and our strengths over the past few years.

In happier times, on a flight home from New York, I read an essay by a rabbi who went to console a man whose wife had died. The rabbi didn't know the man very well, but he stopped off on the way and bought coffee and bagels. In the face of loss, the rabbi reckoned, there was very little he could say, but coffee and bagels are always a good idea.[65]

The rabbi's gesture was small and beautiful. Coffee and bagels signalled connection, care, compassion. Today we need these things more than ever as we lift our Covid-19 restrictions, survey the carnage and figure out what we lost. We lost a lot.

During Covid-19, two features were common to almost every story: loss and resilience. Everyone lost something: a loved one, financial security, a daily routine or a sense of their place in the world.[66] But most stories also tell of resilience, even in the toughest phases of the pandemic. While around one person in five reported significant psychological distress associated with the outbreak, four out of five did not.[67] For many, well-being proved more robust than might have been anticipated.[68] We cope better than we predict we will.

Today, as the pandemic recedes in certain parts of the world, it is important to acknowledge both the strengths and the suffering, and to mourn our losses. For many, what survived is greater than what was lost, but we feel our losses like physical pain. Absence pierces.

In 1969, Swiss-American psychiatrist Elisabeth Kübler-Ross wrote about five stages of grief: denial, anger, bargaining, depression and acceptance.[69] We often deny loss, simply refusing to believe that it has occurred or behaving as if it hasn't. But reality is undeniable, so anger erupts. We bargain with a god we might not believe in. This strategy fails, leading to depression. Ultimately, we accept that life will inexplicably carry on, even in the face of our loss. How can this be?

The stages of grief do not occur in sequence. They come and go. Several stages occur at once. Some never make an appearance. So be it. We cannot negotiate with emotions nor berate them for failing to follow our rules. The heart has a mind of its own.

Despite these complexities, Kübler-Ross's framework is a gift. Her structure provides a language for many aspects of grief. It normalises reactions that might otherwise confuse us. It reassures us that, while individual grief is always unique, other people have walked this path before us. Thousands of people. Millions. Billions—especially after Covid-19.

All of Kübler-Ross's 'stages' have been apparent throughout this pandemic, as the virus moved through our cities and countries with a terrible power that has shaken all of us and broken some of us. Anxiety segued into grief as we understood the magnitude of the outbreak, felt its destructiveness in our bones and—now—see the shape of the world it leaves in its wake. This is a different world, both familiar and unfamiliar at the same time.

How can we cope with this? Are the anxiety and grief too sharp, too pervasive and simply too big for us to handle? Do our weaknesses exceed our strengths? Has Covid-19 broken all of us?

No, not by a long shot. We piece our way through this, using our strengths to circumvent our weaknesses, using insight to resolve doubt.

First, anxiety. During the pandemic, many people realised that they were more prone to anxiety than they imagined, but most also discovered that we are always bigger than our worries. The greater the anxiety, the smaller the steps needed to control it. We followed public health guidance about controlling the virus and found comfort in that. We were doing what we could, adhering to advice.

Clear guidelines were emotionally invaluable. Someone knew what they were doing.

From a psychological perspective, we found strength in managing our intake of media, especially social media, and resisting the siren call of worst-case thinking. It is useful to stay informed but unhelpful to follow every statistic from every country every day. We cannot carry the weight of a global pandemic on our individual shoulders. Enough is enough. Most people learned to detach.

Physical activity helped, as many people discovered that we cannot always think our way out of anxiety. Sometimes we need to shut the laptop, stand up, leave the phone behind and do something. Going outside is magic: it uses our physical strength to address a moment of psychological vulnerability or emotional distress—activity as an antidote to thought. In time, it is addictive.

And what about grief? There are no cures for grief, nor should there be, but time and compassion are powerful salves. Grief passes. Unthinkable as it seems, we find a way to live in our new, different, impoverished world. Recognising feelings of grief helps us to work through them or simply observe them as time passes. There is a Buddhist saying: 'Don't just do something; sit there'. Today we need to sit with grief, our own and that of others.

Compassion is the second salve. Compassion is both a feeling and a skill. We can practise compassion towards ourselves (we are doing our best) and others (so are they). Buddhism speaks of 'non-self', the idea that our 'self' is less concrete than we imagine it to be.[70] Our 'self' changes constantly. We merge into other people all the time.

The spread of Covid-19 and pandemic anxiety demonstrate just how true this is. Humanity functions like a single organism: we live and die together. This is a powerful argument in favour of compassion towards all sentient beings, including ourselves. The suffering of other people is continuous with our suffering, just as their happiness is continuous with ours.

As anxiety turns to grief, our communities will save us.[71] Many communities are sadly smaller but resolutely stronger. When we reflect on the pandemic, there will be pain and coping, loss and survival, crying and singing. And, like before, there will be coffee and bagels. The rabbi was right: symbols matter, coffee works.

Moving outside our own lives and communities, the past few years have demonstrated the weaknesses and strengths of governments around the world. Covid-19 was the first natural disaster to be experienced by this generation in many rich countries. Many poor countries are, tragically, more accustomed to floods, plagues and famines. Even climate change, which touches everyone on the planet, affects poor countries sooner and more.

So, how did governments, rich and poor, cope with Covid-19?

Governments, like individuals, demonstrated a mix of weaknesses and strengths. Initial responses were often panicked, muddled and unhelpful. More could have been done sooner. While the pandemic came as a surprise, reflex responses were still poor. There are no ready comparisons in recent human history, but it should be possible to do better.

Relatively quickly, however, the strengths of governments came into play. It became clear that the power of governments is truly awesome.[72] While private corporations wield considerable economic and political heft, they cannot hold a candle to governments that closed airports, businesses and schools, mounted vast public health responses and then reopened our societies. Only governments can do that.

Power on this scale is breathtaking, so it carries a requirement for openness and accountability, especially with sweeping measures that affect every aspect of our lives. Commenting in *The Guardian* on the UK government's response, Stephen Reicher, Professor of Social Psychology at the University of St Andrews, emphasises the need for transparency:

> Ultimately [...] we need a broader shift in the relationship between the state and its citizens. The government must abandon a psychology that infantilises people. It must recognise and respect the ability of the public to acknowledge and deal with harsh realities. It must engage us as full partners in every stage of the strategy against Covid-19: from formulating a response, to implementing and evaluating policy. And, as in any constructive relationship, none of this can happen without putting openness at the very heart of what government does.[73]

At international level, politicians, like scientists, need to work together, especially when faced with challenges like Covid-19.[74] We need agreed, ongoing measures to protect against new variants: vaccines, face-masks in certain settings and good ventilation (including air filtration).[75] These are small prices to pay to avoid another all-out emergency.

Co-operation is also needed after the pandemic, as its social and economic consequences play out.[76] Xenophobia and hostility towards strangers were often linked with outbreaks in the past; these would be disastrous today.[77] In July 2018, at the Galway International Arts Festival, President Higgins argued that 'solidarity' needs to be inclusive:

> … in the twenty-first century there can be no partial solidarity, whether national solidarity or European solidarity. We require now an international solidarity, shorn of national antagonisms, open and willing to co-operate where we can and sacrifice where we must.[78]

President Higgins adds that 'many of the challenges we confront are those which test our capacity for, and willingness to engage in, collective deliberation to discern the common good, and collective action to achieve it'. Covid-19 adds even greater urgency to President Higgins's calls for 'solidarity' which 'must extend beyond our borders':

> In this precarious world, global solidarity is the most important contribution we can make to peace and stability

[…] Peace cannot be built, nor can it be sustained, by any narrow diplomacy, defined by transaction, in service of a national advantage at the cost of other nations. Peace rests but upon a diplomacy of the common good, one built on mutual respect and understanding, one that is open to the possibilities of the future, one that rejects any invocation of fear.[79]

Despite the suffering inflicted by Covid-19 and its potential impact on solidarity, the pandemic's effect on economies was generally less than expected.[80] The chief social threat is its uneven effect across populations. Covid-19 was never an equal-opportunities virus.[81] It disproportionately affects the poor, minorities and people who are marginalised, as Linda Geddes notes in *The Guardian*:

People living in the UK's most deprived areas are more likely to be infected with Covid-19, but research suggests this relationship is a two-way street: becoming infected also increases people's risk of economic hardship, particularly if they develop long Covid.[82]

Covid-19 offers a unique opportunity to address this kind of social inequality.[83] The weaknesses that it revealed in our societies can be addressed through our strengths and by building solidarity, but this requires sustained political will if it is to last. We owe it to those who died in the pandemic to take whatever good we can from the past few years and build stronger systems to withstand future shocks. Together, we can, with continued monitoring of emerging threats, standing public health response teams and broader steps to address social inequality.

This brings me to the fifth and final lesson that we might or might not learn from this pandemic: the importance of escape.

The past few years have been incredibly intense and filled with questions. What is this new infection? How can we protect our physical and mental health?[84] Were State responses to the virus too brutal?[85] Will young people be psychologically scarred?[86] What might a post-pandemic world look like?[87] Will Covid-19 ever end?[88] Where can we find consolation in the dark times?[89] What is really going on?

These are all valid questions, but many are essentially unanswerable. While it is important that we face these issues, doubts and fears, it is equally important that we set them aside for periods of time and escape into other worlds. We need to think, but we also need to stop thinking. Our minds are too complex to operate at full capacity all the time. We need to switch off.

Even the workaholic Wilde knew this, so he frequently escaped to Moytura, his house near Cong, as well as various other places where he could work if he wished or step back from his concerns if he so desired. We all need a Moytura, a leafy retreat away from the cut and thrust of everyday life, distant from the quiet terrors of the daily grind.

Escape can be mental, physical or—best of all—both.

For those who could not travel far during various phases of the pandemic, there was escape in activities that absorbed us, allowing ourselves to be lost in gardening, running, swimming, knitting or reading, if only for an hour or two. Quiet absorption nourishes the soul. Happiness might be too much to hope for at all times, so it is useful to settle for engrossed quietude and the peace of mind it brings. The world melts away. Absorption allows us to forget our worries. Forgetting is escape. Happiness follows.

In the longer term, what will we remember from Covid-19? It is likely that we will recall details, feelings, personal losses. In time, we will probably forget a great deal of what we think we will remember. We might not learn the five lessons I have outlined here. History might not accord Covid-19 the prominence we feel it merits. In the end, we might remember shockingly little.

In 2019 President Higgins asked: 'Why do some major historical events occupy the forefront of the collective consciousness, while profound moments, such as the [1918 Spanish 'flu] pandemic we are discussing today, sometimes stand distantly behind?'[90] Exploring 'why there is something of a collective amnesia regarding Spanish 'flu', the president pointed to 'limited media coverage' at the time; the fact that 'the general population was familiar with patterns of pandemic disease' during that period in history; and the observation that 'the outbreak coincided with the deaths and media focus on the First World War', and 'the majority of fatalities, from both the War and the epidemic, were among young adults, with the deaths caused by the 'flu potentially overlooked'.

What factors will determine how we remember Covid-19 and what we forget? Should we strive to remember our worries, weaknesses and missteps, in order to learn from them, or should we emphasise our achievements, strengths and solidarity? Do we get to decide this balance or does time decide for us?

I suspect that we will chiefly remember feelings rather than facts, personal events rather than social changes. And yet, despite the suffering, losses and forgetting, and despite the likelihood that we will learn very little for the future, pessimism would be misplaced. We are stronger, smarter and kinder than we think.

In April 1981 Taoiseach Charles Haughey, addressing the National Youth Conference in Dún Laoghaire, said that people should 'not be either intimidated or depressed by the state of the world that you see around you':

> There was no stage in the world's history when the pessimists and the Cassandras could not find ostensible reasons to prophesy final disaster. But they have always been wrong. Despite the great tragedies which have occurred in every age, man perseveres and moves inexorably forward.

Today, as the tragedy of Covid-19 subsides in certain countries, we continue to 'persevere' and move 'inexorably forward'. In May I escape to Wilde's beloved Mayo and climb two mountains, Nephin and Croagh Patrick. This is escape of the highest order that our precious planet has to offer: physical, mental, emotional.

These mountains were big and majestic before Covid-19. After the pandemic they still are. So are we.

EPILOGUE

In late May 2022, I commence my twice-postponed-because-of-Covid-19, twice-rescheduled-because-we-need-to-keep-hope-alive trip to the Camino de Santiago, a pilgrim path in France and Spain.

Almost three years ago, my friend and I planned to walk the 'French Camino', which starts in the town of Saint-Jean-Pied-de-Port on the French side of the Pyrenees and stretches around 800km to the shrine of the apostle Saint James the Great in the cathedral of Santiago de Compostela in north-west Spain.[1] It's a long way, so we plan to make the journey in one-week segments, starting with six days' walking this month.

In preparation, I read about medieval Irish pilgrims on the route,[2] study writer Paulo Coelho's walk in the 1980s,[3] gasp at actress Shirley MacLaine's experiences in 1994[4] and chuckle at Bradley Chermside's recent adventures.[5]

If truth be told, however, my path to this path is chiefly through movies, especially *The Way*, a 2010 film directed by Emilio Estevez.[6] The movie features Martin Sheen as a bereaved father whose son died on the Camino. The film is sentimental but involving.[7] The real star is the path itself. I'm hooked.

In *The Guardian*, Rob Williams noted that the movie's release in 2011 was well-timed:

> In 1985 just 2,500 pilgrims walked to Santiago. Last year [2010], the Confraternity of Saint James reported that more than 150,000 people received their 'compostelas', the certificate of pilgrimage. And interest looks set to increase with the release this month of *The Way* […] the Camino is a fantastic antidote to our stressful lives—and a lesson in deferred gratification. You set little targets, some forced by geography, some self-imposed. So, no water until the top of the hill, no lunch until the next village, nowhere to sleep until the next *refugio*.[8]

I am also weirdly taken with another account of the pilgrimage, a diary kept by German comedian Hape Kerkeling when he travelled the Camino in 2001.[9] Kerkeling gives a very unusual account of the trip, which inspired an even more unusual movie, and I find both oddly compelling.[10] That's it: we're doing the Camino no matter what.

My friend and I stock up on maps and guides.[11] We sit out the Covid-19 pandemic for two full years and then, like all humble pilgrims, start our journey with a flight to Biarritz in May 2022.

I buy extra face-masks for the trip but, three days before we leave, the EU Aviation Safety Agency and the

European Centre for Disease Prevention and Control announce that face-masks will soon no longer be mandatory in airports and on flights in Europe.[12] The new regulations will not be in effect when we fly to Biarritz, but they will be operational when we fly home from Bilbao after (hopefully) walking 130km from Saint-Jean-Pied-de-Port in France to Los Arcos in Spain. We will walk into a freer world.

As we depart from Dublin airport, most people have pre-empted the changes and are not wearing face-masks.[i] When we touch down in Biarritz, even fewer people have their faces covered. As we arrive in Saint-Jean-Pied-de-Port an hour later, only a tiny minority wear a mask. It is as if the pandemic never happened. Wilde, in 1840, described France as a 'brave and enlightened' nation, but I would prefer a little more caution today.[13] The situation has improved, but Covid-19 is not done with us yet.

We stay in a charming hotel in Saint-Jean-Pied-de-Port, where I have the worst night's sleep of my life: nearby music thumps until the early hours, the room is like a sauna and traffic thunders past. I sleep eventually but fitfully. It is a dreadful start.

At breakfast, my friend and I sit in a deserted dining room gazing at a boar's head mounted on the wall. The croissants are delicious.

---

i   I believe this is properly called 'behavioural anticipation' but is more commonly known as 'jumping the gun'.

Why are we walking the Camino? Why now? Our plans pre-dated Covid-19, so while the pandemic gives our trip added meaning it does not explain it fully.

Just over a year ago, in March 2021, Peter Stanford, in *The Observer*, reflected on the upsurge in pilgrims:

> The numbers are striking and puzzling in our secular, sceptical age when organised religion in the west is in steep decline. In the early 1980s, the annual tally of those walking the Camino, the thousand-year-old Christian pilgrim route from France to Santiago de Compostela [...] had dropped to a few thousand at best. By 2019, before Covid got in the way, it was almost 350,000 [...] As we dare this Easter to start making holiday plans again, plenty of pilgrim paths and destinations offer a chance to step back and get a perspective on the trauma we have lived through ...[14]

Stanford is right. This is how we cope. It is how we have always coped. We search for meaning. We walk a path.

After the trials and tribulations, worries and anxieties, losses and bereavements of the past few years, we still find ways to focus on resilience, strength and simply carrying on. Personal traumas evolve, healing happens, societies move forward. The losses are profound, but our survival instinct is strong. We are pilgrims.

As people and societies, Covid-19 taught us that we are more vulnerable than we thought, but also stronger, smarter, wiser and kinder.

As we leave the hotel in Saint-Jean-Pied-de-Port to cross the Pyrenees on Day One of our Camino, the woman behind the desk—the same woman who checked us in, showed us our rooms, gave us our breakfast and checked us out—is cleaning a counter. She looks up and smiles: 'Bon Camino'.

BIBLIOGRAPHY

Adeluwoye, D., 'Mental health problems soar for young people during lockdown', *The Observer*, 30 August 2020.

Ahmad, F.B. and Anderson, R.N., 'The leading causes of death in the US for 2020', *JAMA*, vol. 325 (2021), pp 1829–30 (https://doi.org/10.1001/jama.2021.5469).

Ahuja, A., 'We've had the biggest science policy failure in a generation', *Financial Times*, 25/26 April 2020.

Ahuja, A., 'Lessons on how to live with Covid-19 are still to be learnt', *Financial Times*, 8/9 January 2022.

Arnold, C., *Bedlam: London and its Mad* (London: Simon and Schuster/Pocket Books, 2009).

Beiner, G., Marsh, P. and Milne, I., 'Greatest killer of the twentieth century: the Great Flu of 1918–19', *History Ireland*, vol. 17 (2) (2009), pp 40–3.

Belluck, P., 'Do vaccines protect against long-term Covid symptoms?', *New York Times International Edition*, 28 April 2022.

Bentall, R., 'Has the pandemic really caused a "tsunami" of mental health problems?', *The Guardian*, 9 February 2021.

Bewley, T.H., 'The health of Jonathan Swift', *Journal of the Royal Society of Medicine*, vol. 91 (1998), pp 602–5 (https://doi.org/10.1177/014107689809101118).

Bewley, T.[H.], 'Swift's pocky quean', *Journal of the Royal Society of Medicine*, vol. 92 (1999), p. 216 (https://doi.org/10.1177/014107689909200427).

Bielenberg, K., 'Be alert, but don't be alarmed!', *Irish Independent*, 7 March 2020.

Boland, P. and Hughes, S.P., 'The enigma of Sir William Robert Wills Wilde (1815–1876)', *Journal of Medical Biography*, 21 October 2021 (https://doi.org/10.1177/09677720211046588 [Epub ahead of print]).

Bracken, S., 'Hospital figures for self-harm fall 25%', *Irish Times*, 12 September 2020.

Brain, W.R., 'The illness of Dean Swift', *Irish Journal of Medical Science*, vol. 320–1 (1952), pp 337–45 (https://doi.org/10.1007/BF02956890).

Brennan, D., *Irish Insanity, 1800–2000* (London and New York: Routledge/Taylor and Francis, 2014).

Brennan, M., 'Finding cure for past plagues gives us hope for the future', *Irish Examiner*, 29 April 2022.

Brierley, J., *Camino de Santiago: St. Jean Pied de Port–Santiago de Compostela: Maps* (Dyke: Camino Guides, 2019).

Brooks, S.K., Webster, R.K., Smith, L.E., Woodland, L., Wessely, S., Greenberg, N. and Rubin, G.J., 'The psychological impact of quarantine and how to reduce it: rapid review of the evidence', *The Lancet*, vol. 395

(2020), pp 912–20 (https://doi.org/10.1016/S0140-6736(20)30460-8).

Brown, G., *Seven Ways to Change the World: How to Fix the Most Pressing Problems We Face* (London: Simon and Schuster, 2021).

Burke, T., Berry, A., Taylor, L.K. *et al.*, 'Increased psychological distress during COVID-19 and quarantine in Ireland: a national survey', *Journal of Clinical Medicine*, vol. 9 (2020), E3481 (https://doi.org/10.3390/jcm9113481).

Butler, E., 'Graphic of the week: coffee consumption', *Irish Times*, 17 July 2021.

Camus, A., *La Peste (The Plague)* (Paris: Gallimard, 1947).

Carey, S., 'Personal power to create positive outlook can change paradigm and reduce isolation', *Irish Independent*, 26 February 2022.

Carney, M., *Value(s): Building a Better World for All* (London: William Collins, 2021).

Cavendish, C., 'Britain's youngsters are scarred by post-pandemic anxiety', *Financial Times*, 26/27 February 2022.

Centers for Disease Control and Prevention, *Manage Anxiety and Stress* (Atlanta, GA: Centers for Disease Control and Prevention, 2020).

Chambers, R., *A State of Emergency: The Story of Ireland's Covid Crisis* (Dublin: HarperCollinsIreland, 2021).

Chermisde, B., *The Only Way is West: A Once in a Lifetime Adventure Walking 500 Miles on Spain's Camino de Santiago* (Wrocław: Amazon, 2019).

Chödrön, P., *When Things Fall Apart: Heart Advice for Difficult Times* (Boulder, CO: Shambala Publications, 2016).

Christakis, N.A., *Apollo's Arrow: The Profound and Enduring Impact of Coronavirus on the Way We Live* (New York: Little, Brown Spark, 2020).

Clare, A.W., *A Study of Psychiatric Illness in an Immigrant Irish Population* (MPhil. (Psychiatry) thesis, University of London, 1972).

Clare, A.W., 'Swift, mental illness and St Patrick's Hospital', *Irish Journal of Psychological Medicine*, vol. 15 (1998), pp 100–4 (https://doi.org/10.1017/S0790966700003797).

Coakley, D., *Oscar Wilde: The Importance of Being Irish* (Dublin: Town House, 1994).

Coakley, D., 'William Wilde in the west of Ireland', *Irish Journal of Medical Science*, vol. 185 (2016), pp 277–80 (https://doi.org/10.1007/s11845-016-1433-7).

Coelho, P., *The Pilgrimage: A Contemporary Quest for Ancient Wisdom* (New York: Harper, 2004).

Coleman, C., *News from Under a Coat Stand. A Diary, March–June 2020* (Cork: Orla Kelly Publishing, 2021).

College of Psychiatrists of Ireland, *COVID-19 Impact on Secondary Mental Healthcare Services in Ireland* (Dublin: College of Psychiatrists of Ireland, 2020) (https://www.irishpsychiatry.ie/external-affairs-policy/college-papers-submissions-publications/positions-policies-perspective-papers/covid-19-impact-on-secondary-mental-healthcare-services-in-ireland/).

College of Psychiatrists of Ireland, 'Press Statement', 17 June 2020 (https://www.irishpsychiatry.ie/external-affairs-policy/college-papers-submissions-publications/positions-policies-perspective-papers/covid-19-impact-on-secondary-mental-healthcare-services-in-ireland/).

Collins, S., 'Appointment of Holohan a political molehill', *Irish Times*, 15 April 2022.

Colum, P., *Moytura: A Play for Dancers* (Dublin: Dolmen Press, 1963).

Colvin, C. and McLaughlin, E., 'Revisiting the demography of the 1918 influenza pandemic in Ireland', *History Ireland*, vol. 29 (5) (2021), pp 38–41.

Connell, J., 'Our souls need to catch up after a journey of lockdown before we can savour freedom', *Irish Independent*, 28 January 2022.

Cookson, C., 'Beware fake news, do not panic buy and prepare for possible self-isolation', *Financial Times*, 7/8 March 2020.

Cookson, C., Gross, A., Asgari, N. and Cameron-Chileshe, J., 'How to reach the unvaccinated', *Financial Times*, 12 August 2021.

Cormican, M., 'Ireland's response to the SARS-CoV-2 pandemic. The Marianne Dashwood test', *ResearchGate*, October 2022 (https://www.researchgate.net/publication/365273684_ISCM_COVID_The_Marianne_Dashwood_Test_20102022_M_Cormican).

Corrigan, S., 'No evidence of suicide spike', *Connacht Tribune*, 12 February 2021.

Coto, J., Restrepo, A., Cejas, I. and Prentiss, S., 'The impact of COVID-19 on allied health professions', *PLoS ONE*, vol. 15 (2020), e0241328 (https://doi.org/10.1371/journal.pone.0241328).

COVID-19 Excess Mortality Collaborators, 'Estimating excess mortality due to the COVID-19 pandemic: a systematic analysis of COVID-19-related mortality, 2020–21', *The Lancet*, vol. 399 (2022), pp 1513–36 (https://doi.org/10.1016/S0140-6736(21)02796-3).

Crookes, G., *Dublin's Eye and Ear: The Making of a Monument* (Dublin: Town House, 1993).

Cullen, P., 'Curing our health system from Covid', *Irish Times*, 29 January 2022.

Cullen, P., 'Coronavirus linked to elevated risk of mental health disorders', *Irish Times*, 17 February 2022.

Cullen, P., 'Latest Covid wave catches us off guard', *Irish Times*, 26 March 2022.

Cullen, W., Gulati, G. and Kelly, B.D., 'Mental health in the Covid-19 pandemic', *QJM*, vol. 113 (2020), pp 311–12 (https://doi.org/10.1093/qjmed/hcaa110).

Cunningham, B., *Medieval Irish Pilgrims to Santiago de Compostela* (Dublin: Four Courts Press, 2018).

De Hert, M., Mazereel, V., Detraux, J. and Van Assche, K., 'Prioritizing COVID-19 vaccination for people with severe mental illness', *World Psychiatry*, vol. 20 (2021), pp 54–5 (https://doi.org/10.1002/wps.20826).

de Vere White, T., *The Parents of Oscar Wilde: Sir William and Lady Wilde* (London: Hodder and Stoughton, 1967).

Defalque, R.J. and Wright, A.J., 'Travers vs. Wilde and other: chloroform acquitted', *Bulletin of Anesthesia History*, vol. 23 (1) (2005), pp 4–7 (https://doi.org/10.1016/s1522-8649(05)50045-3).

Donnelly, W. and Wilde, W.R., *The Census of Ireland for the Year 1851, Part III: Report on the Status of Disease* (Dublin: Alexander Thom and Sons, for Her Majesty's Stationery Office, 1854).

Donnelly, W. and Wilde, W.R., *The Census of Ireland for the Year 1851, Part V: Tables of Deaths. Volume I, Containing the Report, Tables of Pestilences, and Analysis of the Tables of Deaths* (Dublin: Alexander Thom and Sons, for Her Majesty's Stationery Office, 1856).

Donnelly, W. and Wilde, W.R., *The Census of Ireland for the Year 1851, Part V: Tables of Deaths. Volume II, Containing the Tables and Index* (Dublin: Alexander Thom and Sons, for Her Majesty's Stationery Office, 1856).

Douaud, G., Lee, S., Alfaro-Almagro, F. *et al.*, 'SARS-CoV-2 is associated with changes in brain structure in UK Biobank', *Nature*, vol. 604 (2022), pp 697–707 (https://doi.org/10.1038/s41586-022-04569-5).

Doyle, A., 'Inquiry into response to Covid pandemic', *Irish Times*, 10 March 2023.

Doyle, K., 'A new beginning', *Irish Independent*, 22 January 2022.

Duan, L. and Zhu, G., 'Psychological interventions for people affected by the COVID-19 epidemic', *Lancet Psychiatry*, vol. 7 (2020), pp 300–2 (https://doi.org/10.1016/S2215-0366(20)30073-0).

Economist, The, 'The big picture', *The Economist*, 2 January 2021.

Economist, The, 'And now for the aftershock', *The Economist*, 1 May 2021.

Economist, The, 'Vaccinating the world', *The Economist*, 15 May 2021.

Economist, The, 'The triumph of big government', *The Economist*, 20 November 2021.

Economist, The, 'The fourth wave', *The Economist*, 27 November 2021.

Economist, The, 'The new normal', *The Economist*, 18 December 2021.

Economist, The, 'Omicron causes a less severe illness than earlier variants', *The Economist*, 1 January 2022.

Economist, The, 'Battling the superbugs', *The Economist*, 22 January 2022.

Efstathiou, V., Stefanou, M.-I., Siafakas, N. *et al.*, 'Suicidality and COVID-19: suicidal ideation, suicidal behaviors and completed suicides amidst the COVID-19 pandemic (review)', *Experimental and Therapeutic Medicine*, vol. 23 (2022), p. 107 (https://doi.org/10.3892/etm.2021.11030).

Ellmann, R., *Oscar Wilde* (New York: Vintage Books, 1988).

Farrar, J. and Ahuja, A., *Spike: The Virus vs the People. The Inside Story* (paperback edn) (London: Profile Books, 2022).

Ferry, G., 'A woman's place. Dorothy Stopford Price and the control of tuberculosis in Ireland', *The Lancet*, vol. 393 (2019), p. 20 (https://doi.org/10.1016/S0140-6736(18)33171-4).

Finnerty, S., *Physical Health of People with Severe Mental Illness* (Dublin: Mental Health Commission, 2019) (https://www.mhcirl.ie/publications/physical-health-people-severe-mental-illness).

Fitzpatrick, C., *Poetic Licence in a Time of Corona* (Dublin: Twenty First Century Renaissance, 2022).

Foley, C., *The Last Irish Plague: The Great Flu Epidemic in Ireland, 1918–19* (Dublin and Portland, OR: Irish Academic Press, 2011).

Foley, S.J., O'Loughlin, A. and Creedon, J., 'Early experiences of radiographers in Ireland during the COVID-19 crisis', *Insights into Imaging*, vol. 11 (2020), p. 104 (https://doi.org/10.1186/s13244-020-00910-6).

Foster, R., 'Sins of the fathers', *The Spectator*, 15 December 2018.

Freeman, L., 'A year of Covid lessons from a monk's cloistered cell', *Financial Times*, 3/4 April 2021.

French, P., '*The Way*—review', *The Observer*, 15 May 2011 (https://www.theguardian.com/film/2011/may/15/the-way-emilio-estevez-martin-sheen-review).

Freud, E. (ed.), *Letters of Sigmund Freud, Selected and Edited by Ernst Freud, 1873–1939* (New York: Dover Publications, 1960).

Freud, S., 'Delusions and Dreams in Jensen's *Gradiva* (1906/7)', in *The Standard Edition of the Complete Psychological Works of Sigmund Freud, Volume IX (1906–*

1908) (London: Vintage, Hogarth Press and Institute of Psycho-Analysis, 2001).

Freud, S., 'Civilization and its Discontents (1929/30)', in *The Standard Edition of the Complete Psychological Works of Sigmund Freud, Volume XXI (1927–1931)* (London: Vintage, Hogarth Press and Institute of Psycho-Analysis, 2001).

Froggatt, P., 'Sir William Wilde and the 1851 Census of Ireland', *Medical History*, vol. 9 (1965), pp 302–27 (https://doi.org/10.1017/s0025727300030970).

Froggatt, P., 'Sir William Wilde, 1815–1876. A centenary appreciation: Wilde's place in medicine', *Proceedings of the Royal Irish Academy*, vol. 77C (1977), pp 261–78.

Froggatt, P., 'The demographic work of Sir William Wilde', *Irish Journal of Medical Science*, vol. 185 (2016), pp 293–5 (https://doi.org/10.1007/s11845-016-1436-4).

Fujiwara, D., Dolan, P., Lawton, R., Behzadnejad, F., Lagarde, A., Maxwell, C. and Peytrignet, S., *The Wellbeing Costs of COVID-19 in the UK: An Independent Research Report by Simetrica-Jacobs and the London School of Economics and Political Science* (London: Simetrica-Jacobs and the London School of Economics and Political Science, 2020) (https://www.lse.ac.uk/News/Latest-news-from-LSE/2020/e-May-20/Wellbeing-and-COVID-19).

Galloway, S., *Post Corona: From Crisis to Opportunity* (London: Bantam Press, 2020).

Ganesh, J., 'Resist a false divination from the Covid crisis', *Financial Times*, 30 December 2020.

García-Álvarez, L., de la Fuente-Tomás, L., García-Portilla, M.P. *et al.*, 'Early psychological impact of the 2019 coronavirus disease (COVID-19) pandemic and lockdown in a large Spanish sample', *Journal of Global Health*, vol. 10 (2020), 020505 (https://doi.org/10.7189/jogh.10.020505).

Gates, B., *How to Prevent the Next Pandemic* (London: Allen Lane, 2022).

Gavin, B., Hayden, J., Adamis, D. and McNicholas, F., 'Caring for the psychological well-being of healthcare professionals in the Covid-19 pandemic crisis', *Irish Medical Journal*, vol. 113 (2020), pp 51–3 (http://imj.ie/caring-for-the-psychological-well-being-of-front-line-workers-during-covid-19/).

Geary, L., 'William Wilde: historian', *Irish Journal of Medical Science*, vol. 185 (2016), pp 301–2 (https://doi.org/10.1007/s11845-016-1427-5).

Geddes, L., 'Having Covid-19 linked to risk of economic hardship, study suggests', *The Guardian*, 9 March 2022 (https://www.theguardian.com/society/2022/mar/09/covid-19-risk-economic-hardship-poverty-study-suggests).

Gilligan, P., 'Chief Executive's Foreword', in *St Patrick's Mental Health Services Annual Report and Financial Statements 2020* (Dublin: St Patrick's Mental Health Services, 2021), pp 4–5 (https://www.stpatricks.ie/media-centre/news/2021/july/annualandoutcomesreport2020).

Glynn, R., 'Think of vaccination as an added safety feature against Covid', *Irish Examiner*, 13 August 2021.

Graham-Harrison, E., 'China sticks to zero Covid policy—but how long can isolation last?', *The Observer*, 2 January 2022 (https://www.theguardian.com/world/2022/jan/01/china-zero-covid-strategy-beijing-policy-protecting-public-health-coronavirus [courtesy of *Guardian* News & Media Ltd]).

Gross, A., 'History shows pandemics rarely end neatly or with complete eradication', *Financial Times*, 13/14 March 2021.

Guardian, The, '*The Guardian* view on tackling the new coronavirus: handle with care: editorial', *The Guardian*, 7 February 2020 (https://www.theguardian.com/commentisfree/2020/feb/07/the-guardian-view-on-tackling-the-new-coronavirus-handle-with-care).

Gulati, G. and Kelly, B.D., 'Domestic violence against women and the Covid-19 pandemic: what is the role of psychiatry?', *International Journal of Law and Psychiatry*, vol. 71 (2020), p. 101594 (https://doi.org/10.1016/j.ijlp.2020.101594).

Gulati, G. and Kelly, B.D., 'Physician suicide and the COVID-19 pandemic', *Occupational Medicine*, vol. 70 (2020), p. 514 (https://doi.org/10.1093/occmed/kqaa104).

Gulati, G., Dunne, C.P. and Kelly, B.D., 'Do COVID-19 responses imperil the human rights of people with disabilities?', *Health and Human Rights Journal*, 3 June 2020 (https://www.hhrjournal.org/2020/06/do-covid-19-responses-imperil-the-human-rights-of-people-with-disabilities/).

Gulati, G., Kelly, B.D., Dunne, C.P. and Glynn, L., 'Rise in violence in general practice settings during the COVID-19 pandemic: implications for prevention', *Family Practice*, vol. 38 (2021), pp 696–8 (https://doi.org/10.1093/fampra/cmab060).

Guo, Q., Zheng, Y., Shi, J. *et al.*, 'Immediate psychological distress in quarantined patients with COVID-19 and its association with peripheral inflammation: a mixed-method study', *Brain, Behavior, and Immunity*, vol. 88 (2020), pp 17–27 (https://doi.org/10.1016/j.bbi.2020.05.038).

Hanberry, G., *More Lives Than One: The Remarkable Wilde Family through the Generations* (Cork: Collins Press, 2011).

Harari, Y.N., 'The world after coronavirus', *Financial Times*, 21/22 March 2020.

Harari, Y.N., 'The Covid year', *Financial Times*, 27/28 February 2021.

Harding, R., 'Human progress stumbles on, Covid or no Covid', *Financial Times*, 22 December 2021.

Harford, T., 'Falsehoods spread and mutate just like a virus', *Financial Times*, 7/8 March 2020.

Harrold, P., 'Burned out GPs boosted from giving first round of jabs', *Irish Times*, 23 March 2021.

Hayhoe, K., *Saving Us: A Climate Scientist's Case for Hope and Healing in a Divided World* (New York: One Signal Publishers/Atria, 2021).

Healthy Ireland, Department of Health, Health Service Executive and National Office for Suicide Prevention,

Connecting for Life: Ireland's National Strategy to Reduce Suicide, 2015–2020 (Dublin: Department of Health, 2015) (http://health.gov.ie/wp-content/uploads/2015/06/Connecting-for-Life_LR.pdf).

Hellewell, J., Abbott, S., Gimma, A. *et al.*, 'Feasibility of controlling COVID-19 outbreaks by isolation of cases and contacts', *Lancet Global Health*, vol. 8 (2020), e488–96 (https://doi.org/10.1016/S2214-109X(20)30074-7).

Henderson, R., *Reimagining Capitalism in a World on Fire* (London: Penguin Business, 2021).

Henley, J. and Oltermann, P., 'Why is Europe returning to the dark days of Covid?', *The Observer*, 14 November 2021 (https://www.theguardian.com/world/2021/nov/13/why-is-europe-returning-to-the-dark-days-of-covid [courtesy of *Guardian* News & Media Ltd]).

Henry, C., 'Covid-19 is not just affecting our bodies—it's also getting us down', *Irish Medical Times*, 10 November 2021.

Higgins, R.A., *Pathogens Love a Patsy: Pandemic and Other Poems* (Cliffs of Moher: Salmon Poetry, 2020).

Higgins, V., Sohaei, D., Diamandis, E.P. and Prassas, I., 'COVID-19: from an acute to chronic disease? Potential long-term health consequences', *Critical Reviews in Clinical Laboratory Sciences*, vol. 58 (2021), pp 297–310 (https://doi.org/10.1080/10408363.2020.1860895).

Hitzeroth, V. and Lavelle, I., 'Looking after the medics during the pandemic', *Irish Medical Times*, vol. 55 (2021), p. 16.

Holland, K., 'Suicides have not increased in past year, figures show', *Irish Times*, 2 March 2021.

Honigsbaum, M., 'The art of medicine. Spanish influenza redux: revisiting the mother of all pandemics', *The Lancet*, vol. 391 (2018), pp 2492–5 (https://doi.org/10.1016/S0140-6736(18)31360-6).

Honigsbaum, M., *The Pandemic Century: One Hundred Years of Panic, Hysteria and Hubris* (London: C. Hurst, 2019).

Honigsbaum, M., 'The silent killer we should have seen coming', *The Observer*, 21 June 2020.

Horgan-Jones, J. and O'Connell, H., *Pandemonium: Power, Politics and Ireland's Pandemic* (Dublin: Gill Books, 2022).

Horton, R., *The Covid-19 Catastrophe: What's Gone Wrong and How to Stop it Happening Again* (Cambridge: Polity Press, 2020).

Hossain, M.M., Tasnim, S., Sultana, A. *et al.*, 'Epidemiology of mental health problems in COVID-19: a review', *F1000Research*, vol. 9 (2020), p. 636 (https://doi.org/10.12688/f1000research.24457.1).

Houston, M., 'Covid-19 and its effects on our mental health', *Irish Times*, 15 June 2021.

Houston, M., 'Do we need to reassess our confidence in Covid vaccine?', *Irish Times*, 2 November 2021.

HSE National Office for Suicide Prevention, *Annual Report 2019* (Dublin: Health Service Executive, 2020) (https://www.hse.ie/eng/services/list/4/mental-health-services/

connecting-for-life/publications/nosp-annual-re-port-2019.pdf).

Hunt, J., 'The future of work', *Irish Times*, 23 April 2022.

Huremović, D. (ed.), *Psychiatry of Pandemics: A Mental Health Response to Infection Outbreak* (Cham: Springer, 2019).

Hutton, W., 'Coronavirus won't end globalisation, but change it hugely for the better', *The Observer*, 8 March 2020 (https://www.theguardian.com/commentisfree/2020/mar/08/the-coronavirus-outbreak-shows-us-that-no-one-can-take-on-this-enemy-alone).

Hyland, P., Vallières, F., Shevlin, M., Murphy, J., McBride, O., Karatzias, T. and Bentall, R., *COVID-19 mental health survey by Maynooth University and Trinity College finds high rates of anxiety* (Maynooth: Maynooth University, 2020) (https://www.maynoothuniversity.ie/news-events/covid-19-mental-health-survey-maynooth-university-and-trinity-college-finds-high-rates-anxiety).

Ignatieff, M., *On Consolation: Finding Solace in Dark Times* (New York: Metropolitan Books, 2021).

Irish Times, 'Ireland's Covid restrictions now second lightest in the world', *Irish Times*, 27 March 2022.

Ivanišević, M., 'Albrecht von Graefe's ophthalmic educational visit to William Wilde in Dublin in 1851', *Irish Medical Journal*, vol. 113 (2020), p. 24 (http://imj.ie/albrecht-von-graefes-ophthalmic-educational-visit-to-william-wilde-in-dublin-in-1851/).

Jenkins, S., 'Let them wash your hands, but not your brain', *The Guardian*, 7 March 2020.

Jenkins, S., 'Was I wrong? Even scientists still don't agree on Covid-19', *The Guardian*, 3 April 2020 (https://www.theguardian.com/commentisfree/2020/apr/02/wrong-coronavirus-world-scientists-optimism-experts).

Jones, T., 'The rebirth of humanity', *The Observer*, 12 April 2020 (https://www.theguardian.com/world/2020/apr/12/after-coronavirus-the-penny-has-dropped-that-wellbeing-isnt-individual-but-social).

Joyce, M., Arensman, E. and Griffin, E., 'No visible increase in suicides in pandemic', *Irish Examiner*, 30 April 2021.

Kelly, B.D., *Custody, Care and Criminality: Forensic Psychiatry and Law in 19th Century Ireland* (Dublin: History Press Ireland, 2014).

Kelly, B.D., *Hearing Voices: The History of Psychiatry in Ireland* (Dublin: Irish Academic Press, 2016).

Kelly, B.D., 'Are we finally making progress with suicide and self-harm? An overview of the history, epidemiology and evidence for prevention', *Irish Journal of Psychological Medicine*, vol. 35 (2018), pp 95–101 (https://doi.org/10.1017/ipm.2017.51).

Kelly, B.D., *The Doctor Who Sat for a Year* (Dublin: Gill Books, 2019).

Kelly, B.D., 'Panic and hysteria will only weaken effort to halt virus', *Irish Times*, 2 March 2020 (https://www.irishtimes.com/opinion/panic-and-hysteria-will-undermine-efforts-to-contain-coronavirus-1.4189459).

Kelly, B.D., 'Coronavirus: should we keep calm and carry on?', *The Guardian*, 9 March 2020.

Kelly, B.D., 'We're all in an emotionally complex position—sharing our fears with others helps', *Irish Independent*, 24 March 2020 (https://www.independent.ie/opinion/comment/were-all-in-an-emotionally-complex-position-sharing-our-fears-with-others-helps-39070543.html).

Kelly, B.D., 'Coping with coronavirus: if you want to be heard, listen (Blogpost)', *Psychology Today*, 25 March 2020 (https://www.psychologytoday.com/ie/blog/psychiatry-and-society/202003/coping-coronavirus-if-you-want-be-heard-listen [© Brendan Kelly]).

Kelly, B.D., 'Giving thanks in the time of Covid-19 (Blogpost)', *Psychology Today*, 25 April 2020 (https://www.psychologytoday.com/ie/blog/psychiatry-and-society/202004/giving-thanks-in-the-time-covid-19 [© Brendan Kelly]).

Kelly, B.D., 'Covid-19 and mental illness', *Irish Times*, 27 April 2020.

Kelly, B.D., 'The spread of disease is always political but then so is the cure', *Financial Times*, 2/3 May 2020.

Kelly, B.D., 'Tenacity of the human spirit', *Irish Times*, 12 May 2020.

Kelly, B.D., 'What we've lost, how we'll recover (Blogpost)', *Psychology Today*, 20 May 2020 (https://www.psychologytoday.com/ie/blog/psychiatry-and-society/202005/what-weve-lost-how-well-recover [© Brendan Kelly]).

Kelly, B.D., 'Mind your mental health during this most psychologically difficult phase of the pandemic', *Irish Independent*, 25 August 2020.

Kelly, B.D., 'Coronavirus disease: challenges for psychiatry', *British Journal of Psychiatry*, vol. 217 (2020), pp 352–3 (https://doi.org/10.1192/bjp.2020.86).

Kelly, B.D., *Coping with Coronavirus. How to Stay Calm and Protect Your Mental Health: A Psychological Toolkit* (Newbridge: Merrion Press, 2020).

Kelly, B.D., 'Plagues, pandemics and epidemics in Irish history prior to COVID-19 (coronavirus): what can we learn?', *Irish Journal of Psychological Medicine*, vol. 37 (2020), pp 269–74 (https://doi.org/10.1017/ipm.2020.25).

Kelly, B.D., 'Between hope and despair, we must try to hold the line in the face of the coronavirus', *Irish Independent*, 31 October 2020.

Kelly, B.D., 'COVID-19: real problems but no pandemic of mental illness (Blogpost)', *Psychology Today*, 17 November 2020 (https://www.psychologytoday.com/ie/blog/psychiatry-and-society/202011/covid-19-real-problems-no-pandemic-mental-illness [© Brendan Kelly]).

Kelly, B.D., 'Politicians are as important as doctors for Covid recovery', *Sunday Times*, 22 November 2020.

Kelly, B.D., 'Covid-19 and mental health', *Irish Times*, 26 November 2020.

Kelly, B.D., 'Mental health and Covid-19: what can we do?', *Irish Pharmacy News*, November 2020.

Kelly, B.D., 'Impact of Covid-19 on mental health in Ireland: evidence to date', *Irish Medical Journal*, vol. 113 (2020), pp 214–17 (http://imj.ie/impact-of-covid-19-on-mental-health-in-ireland-evidence-to-date/).

Kelly, B.D., 'Coping with coronavirus: how to stay calm and protect your mental health (Blogpost)', *Lust for Life*, 19 January 2021 (https://www.alustforlife.com/tools/coping-with-coronavirus-how-to-stay-calm-and-protect-your-mental-health).

Kelly, B.D., 'Vaccination is what makes this lockdown different to the last one', *The Echo Newspaper, Tallaght*, 21 January 2021 (https://www.echo.ie/vaccination-is-what-makes-this-lockdown-different-to-the-last-one/).

Kelly, B.D., 'The five stages of Covid's psychological impact', *Irish Independent*, 27 February 2021.

Kelly, B.D., 'Despite all that's going wrong in the world, we are still a pretty happy bunch', *Irish Independent*, 1 April 2021.

Kelly, B.D., 'Pandemic is unfair, not NPHET or the government', *Irish Times*, 13 July 2021.

Kelly, B.D., 'Quarantine, restrictions and mental health in the COVID-19 pandemic', *QJM*, vol. 114 (2021), pp 93–4 (https://doi.org/10.1093/qjmed/hcaa322).

Kelly, B.D., 'The effects of the Covid-19 pandemic on suicide and self-harm', *Update: Psychiatry and Neurology*, vol. 7 (2021), pp 20–1.

Kelly, B.D., 'How to protect your mental health during the Covid-19 pandemic', *Update: Psychiatry and Neurology*, vol. 7 (2021), pp 26–7.

Kelly, B.D., 'Pandemics and the lessons of history', *Irish Times*, 14 August 2021 (https://www.irishtimes.com/opinion/letters/pandemics-and-the-lessons-of-history-1.4646534).

Kelly, B.D., *The Science of Happiness: The Six Principles of a Happy Life and the Seven Strategies for Achieving it* (Dublin: Gill Books, 2021).

Kelly, B.D., 'What does being Irish mean to me?', in M.-C. Logue (ed.), *Being Irish: 101 Views on Irish Identity Today* (Dublin: The Liffey Press, 2021), pp 128–30.

Kelly, B.D., 'The woman who shot Mussolini', *Medical Independent*, 27 January 2022.

Kelly, B.D., 'Kay proves again why he is publishing's gain and medicine's loss', *Medical Independent*, 16 December 2022 (https://www.medicalindependent.ie/life/book-review/kay-proves-again-why-he-is-publishings-gain-and-medicines-loss/).

Kelly, B.D., 'Coffee, travel, and Sir William Wilde', *Medical Independent*, 7 February 2023 (https://www.medicalindependent.ie/comment/opinion/coffee-travel-and-sir-william-wilde/).

Kelly, B.D. and Gulati, G., 'The psychiatric impact of post-Covid-19 syndrome', *Update: Psychiatry and Neurology*, vol. 8 (2022), pp 34–5.

Kelly, B.D. and Gulati, G., 'The psychiatric impact of post-Covid-19 syndrome', *Medical Independent*, 24 February 2022 (https://www.medicalindependent.ie/clinical-news/psychiatry/the-psychiatric-impact-of-post-covid-19-syndrome/).

Kelly, B.D. and Gulati, G., 'Long COVID: the elephant in the room', *QJM*, vol. 115 (2022), pp 5–6 (https://doi.org/10.1093/qjmed/hcab299).

Kelly, B.D. and Houston, M., *Psychiatrist in the Chair: The Official Biography of Anthony Clare* (Dublin: Merrion Press, 2020).

Kelly, I., 'Many lessons in public health learned this year', *Irish Examiner*, 19 April 2021.

Kempton, B., *Wabi Sabi: Japanese Wisdom for a Perfectly Imperfect Life* (London: Piatkus, 2018).

Kerkeling, H., *I'm Off Then: Losing and Finding Myself on the Camino de Santiago* (New York: Free Press, 2009).

Khraisat, B., Toubasi, A., AlZoubi, L., Al-Sayegh, T. and Mansour, A., 'Meta-analysis of prevalence: the psychological sequelae among COVID-19 survivors', *International Journal of Psychiatry in Clinical Practice*, vol. 26 (2022), pp 234–43 (https://doi.org/10.1080/13651501.2021.1993924).

Kirkpatrick, T.P.C., *A Note on the History of the Care of the Insane in Ireland up to the End of the Nineteenth Century* (Dublin: University Press/Ponsonby and Gibbs, 1931).

Kirkpatrick, T.P.C., 'Obituary: Richard Robert Leeper', *Journal of Mental Science*, vol. 88 (1942), pp 480–1 (https://doi.org/10.1192/bjp.88.372.480).

Kübler-Ross, E., *On Death and Dying* (New York: Macmillan, 1969).

Kuchler, H., 'Scientists battle to see off long Covid crisis', *Financial Times*, 5 January 2022.

Lai, J., Ma, S., Wang, Y. *et al.*, 'Factors associated with mental health outcomes among health care workers exposed to coronavirus disease 2019', *JAMA Network*

Open, vol. 3 (2020), e203976 (https://doi.org/10.1001/ jamanetworkopen.2020.3976).

Lancet, The, 'COVID-19: fighting panic with information', *The Lancet*, vol. 395 (2020), p. 537 (https://doi. org/10.1016/S0140-6736(20)30379-2).

Lancet, The, 'COVID-19: too little, too late?', *The Lancet*, vol. 395 (2020), p. 755 (https://doi.org/10.1016/S0140- 6736(20)30522-5).

Lancet, The, 'Facing up to long COVID', *The Lancet*, vol. 396 (2020), p. 1861 (https://doi.org/10.1016/S0140- 6736(20)32662-3).

Leahy, P., Horgan-Jones, J. and McQuinn, C., 'Emergency over', *Irish Times*, 22 and 23 January 2022.

Lee, C., 'Chairman's opening address at the Sir William Wilde bi-centenary symposium', *Irish Journal of Medical Science*, vol. 185 (2016), pp 275–6 (https://doi. org/10.1007/s11845-016-1432-8).

Levin, B., 'The questions machines cannot answer', *The Times*, 3 October 1978.

Levine, H.B. and de Staal, A. (eds), *Psychoanalysis and Covidian Life: Common Distress, Individual Experience* (Bicester: Phoenix, 2021).

Lévy, B.-H., *The Virus in the Age of Madness* (New Haven and London: Yale University Press, 2020).

Lewis, M., *The Premonition: A Pandemic Story* (London: Allen Lane, 2021).

Lou, E., *Field Notes from a Pandemic: A Journey through a World Suspended* (Toronto: Signal/McClelland and Stewart/Penguin Random House Canada, 2020).

Lynch, D., 'Drinking patterns in the pandemic', *Medical Independent*, 27 January 2022.

Lyons, J.B., 'Sir William Wilde's medico-legal observations', *Medical History*, vol. 42 (1997), pp 437–54 (https://doi.org/10.1017/s0025727300063031).

McCarrick, C., Gribben, A. and Lyons, D., 'To have and to hold: repercussions of lockdown in psychiatry', *Hospital Doctor of Ireland*, vol. 27 (2021), pp 25–8.

McCarthy, M., 'Working from home has its benefits—but we badly miss that daily human connection', *Irish Independent*, 31 August 2021.

McCarthy, M., 'As soon as we get the official nod to ditch the masks, I will be ripping mine off', *Irish Independent*, 19 February 2022.

McCarthy, M., 'Learning to roll with the disappointments will make travel and holidays much easier', *Irish Independent*, 2 June 2022.

McEntegart, R., 'William Wilde and 1 Merrion Square', *Irish Journal of Medical Science*, vol. 185 (2016), pp 285–9 (https://doi.org/10.1007/s11845-016-1423-9).

McGeachie, J., 'Wilde's worlds: Sir William Wilde in Victorian Ireland', *Irish Journal of Medical Science*, vol. 185 (2016), pp 303–7 (https://doi.org/10.1007/s11845-016-1428-4).

McGee, H., 'Estimated 114,000 may suffer long Covid', *Irish Times*, 28 January 2022.

McIntyre, A., Tong, K., McMahon, E. and Doherty, A.M., 'COVID-19 and its effect on emergency presentations to a tertiary hospital with self-harm in Ireland', *Irish Journal of Psychological Medicine*, vol. 38 (2021), pp 116–22 (https://doi.org/10.1017/ipm.2020.116).

MacKenzie, D., *Stopping the Next Pandemic: How Covid-19 Can Help Us Save Humanity* (London: Bridge Street Press, 2020).

MacLaine, S., *The Camino: A Pilgrimage of Courage* (London: Pocket Books, 2001).

Mac Lellan, A., *Dorothy Stopford Price: Rebel Doctor* (Dublin: Irish Academic Press, 2014).

McLysaght, E., 'Please stop acting as if liking coffee is a personality trait', *Irish Times,* 11 September 2021.

McNicholas, F. and Moore, K., 'Covid-19, child and adolescent mental health services (CAMHS) and crises', *Irish Medical Journal,* vol. 115 (2022), p. 522 (http://imj.ie/covid-19-child-adolescent-mental-health-services-camhs-and-crises/).

McWilliams, D., 'We are entering the Roaring Twenties', *Irish Times*, 31 July 2021.

Mahase, E., 'Covid-19: what do we know about "long covid"?', *BMJ*, vol. 370 (2020), m2815 (https://doi.org/10.1136/bmj.m2815).

Mak, I.W.C., Chu, C.M., Pan, P.C., Yiu, M.G.C. and Chan, V.L., 'Long-term psychiatric morbidities among SARS survivors', *General Hospital Psychiatry*, vol. 31 (2009), pp 318–26 (https://doi.org/10.1016/j.genhosppsych.2009.03.001).

Malcolm, E., *Swift's Hospital: A History of St Patrick's Hospital, Dublin, 1746–1989* (Dublin: Gill and Macmillan, 1989).

Mance, H., 'A shock to the system', *Financial Times*, 7/8 March 2020.

Mance, H., 'Happiness can still be found during the crisis', *Financial Times*, 30/31 January 2021.

Marshall, M., 'How can we end the pandemic?', *New Scientist*, vol. 253 (2022), pp 12–15.

Meagher, J., 'Generation Precarious: no security in work, at home or for old age', *Irish Independent*, 17 July 2021.

Mills, K., 'Emergence of new variant adds to urgency of booster campaign', *Irish Times*, 27 November 2021.

Milne, I., *Stacking the Coffins: Influenza, War and Revolution in Ireland, 1918–19* (Manchester: Manchester University Press, 2018).

Milne, I., 'Learning from the past', *Irish Examiner*, 13 March 2020.

Minihan, E., Gavin, B., Kelly, B.D. and McNicholas, F., 'COVID-19, mental health and psychological first aid', *Irish Journal of Psychological Medicine*, vol. 37 (2020), pp 259–63 (https://doi.org/10.1017/ipm.2020.41).

Moreno-Pérez, O., Merino, E., Leon-Ramirez, J.-M. *et al.*, 'Post-acute COVID-19 syndrome. Incidence and risk factors: a Mediterranean cohort study', *Journal of Infection*, vol. 82 (2021), pp 373–8 (https://doi.org/10.1016/j.jinf.2021.01.004).

Moriarty, J., *Dreamtime* (Dublin: Lilliput Press, 1994).

Mullaney, S., 'Sir William Wilde and provision for the blind in nineteenth-century Ireland', *Irish Journal of Medical Science*, vol. 185 (2016), pp 281–3 (https://doi.org/10.1007/s11845-016-1434-6).

Murphy, C., 'Can we stop "living" Covid morning, noon and night—and just live with it?', *Sunday Independent*, 28 November 2021.

Murphy, C., 'Pandemic arguments echo through the ages', *Sunday Independent*, 1 May 2022.

Murphy, C., 'Never forget—Covid inquiry must repair brain fog caused by ditching our values', *Sunday Independent*, 19 March 2023.

Naghavi, M., on behalf of the Global Burden of Disease Self-Harm Collaborators, 'Global, regional, and national burden of suicide mortality 1990 to 2016: systematic analysis for the Global Burden of Disease Study 2016', *BMJ*, vol. 364 (2019), p. 194 (https://doi.org/10.1136/bmj.194).

National Institute for Health and Care Excellence (NICE), Scottish Intercollegiate Guidelines Network (SIGN) and Royal College of General Practitioners (RCGP), *COVID-19 Rapid Guideline: Managing the Long-Term Effects of COVID-19* (London: NICE, 2021).

Naughton, J., 'How a global health crisis turns into a state-run surveillance opportunity', *The Observer*, 8 March 2020.

Neylon, L., 'In Phibsborough, a park that's always been locked may soon open', *Dublin Inquirer*, April 2022.

O'Brien, L., 'The magic wisp: a history of the mentally ill in Ireland', *Bulletin of the Menninger Clinic*, vol. 31 (1967), pp 79–95.

O'Connell, J., 'Covid has taught our health system nothing', *Irish Times*, 26 March 2022.

O'Connor, K., Wrigley, M., Jennings, R., Hill, M. and Niazi, A., 'Mental health impacts of COVID-19 in Ireland and the need for a secondary care mental health service response', *Irish Journal of Psychological Medicine*, vol. 38 (2021), pp 99–107 (https://doi.org/10.1017/ipm.2020.64).

O'Doherty, M., 'Sir William Wilde: an enlightened editor', *Irish Journal of Medical Science*, vol. 185 (2016), pp 297–9 (https://doi.org/10.1007/s11845-016-1437-3).

O'Hagan, S., 'The psychological cost of Covid-19', *The Observer*, 7 June 2020 (https://www.theguardian.com/world/2020/jun/07/health-experts-on-the-psychological-cost-of-covid-19 [courtesy of *Guardian* News & Media Ltd]).

O'Leary, N., 'Is this the end of the pandemic?', *Irish Times*, 12 February 2022.

O'Malley, E., 'Broadcast media obsession with daily Covid stats is self-serving', *Sunday Independent*, 28 November 2021.

O'Neill, L., *Keep Calm and Trust the Science: An Extraordinary Year in the Life of an Immunologist* (Dublin: Gill Books, 2021).

O'Regan, E., 'Suggestion 114,500 people have long Covid is an "underestimate"', *Irish Independent*, 29 January 2022.

O'Regan, E., 'Covid-19 impact below EU average', *Irish Examiner*, 8 April 2022.

O'Sullivan, E., *The Fall of the House of Wilde* (London: Bloomsbury, 2016).

Ord, T., 'The importance of worst-case thinking', *The Guardian*, 6 March 2020.

Paul, M., 'Government didn't do enough to stop this surge', *Irish Times*, 19 November 2021.

Paul, M., 'Good riddance to the Covid restrictions', *Irish Times*, 4 February 2022.

Peckham, R., 'COVID-19 and the anti-lessons of history', *The Lancet*, vol. 395 (2020), pp 850–2 (https://doi.org/10.1016/S0140-6736(20)30468-2).

Quinn, B., 'Covid-19 deaths among the fully vaccinated represent just 1.2% of total in England', *The Guardian*, 14 September 2021 (https://www.theguardian.com/world/2021/sep/13/fully-vaccinated-people-account-for-12-of-englands-covid-19-deaths [courtesy of *Guardian* News & Media Ltd]).

Rajan, A. (ed.), *Rethink: Leading Voices on Life After Crisis and How We Can Make a Better World* (London: BBC Books, 2021).

Ramis, S., *Camino de Santiago (Revised and Updated)* (London: Aurum Press, 2017).

Razai, M.S., Doerholt, K., Ladhani, S. and Oakeshott, P., 'Coronavirus disease 2019 (covid-19): a guide for UK GPs', *BMJ*, vol. 368 (2020), m800 (https://doi.org/10.1136/bmj.m800).

Reicher, S., 'No. 10's opacity is corrosive. We need openness', *The Guardian*, 13 May 2020 (https://www.theguardian.com/commentisfree/2020/may/13/british-people-lockdown-coronavirus-crisis).

Robins, J., *Fools and Mad: A History of the Insane in Ireland* (Dublin: Institute of Public Administration, 1986).

Robins, J., *The Miasma: Epidemic and Panic in Nineteenth Century Ireland* (Dublin: Institute of Public Administration, 1995).

Rodgers, M., Dalton, J., Harden, M., Street, A., Parker, G. and Eastwood, A., 'Integrated care to address the physical health needs of people with severe mental illness: a mapping review of the recent evidence on barriers, facilitators and evaluations', *International Journal of Integrated Care*, vol. 18 (2018), p. 9 (https://doi.org/10.5334/ijic.2605).

Sample, I., 'Covid's impact on mental health will last years, royal college warns', *The Guardian*, 28 December 2020.

Scriven, M., Geary, E. and Kelly, B.D., 'Psychiatrists and COVID-19: what is our role during this unprecedented time?', *Irish Journal of Psychological Medicine*, vol. 38 (2021), pp 307–12 (https://doi.org/10.1017/ipm.2020.95).

Shafak, E., *How to Stay Sane in an Age of Division* (London: Profile Books and Wellcome Collection, 2020).

Sontag, S., *Illness as Metaphor* (New York: Farrar, Straus and Giroux, 1978).

Speakman, H., *Here's Ireland* (London: Arrowsmith, 1926).

Spiegelhalter, D. and Masters, A., *Covid by Numbers: Making Sense of the Pandemic with Data* (London: Pelican Books, 2021).

Spiegelhalter, D. and Masters, A., 'Can you capture the complex reality of the pandemic with numbers? Well, we tried …', *The Observer*, 2 January 2022 (https://www.theguardian.com/commentisfree/2022/

jan/02/2021-year-when-interpreting-covid-statistics-crucial-to-reach-truth).

Spinney, L., '"We must revive the social state". Pandemics can lead to equality, suggests Piketty', *The Guardian*, 13 May 2020 (https://www.theguardian.com/world/2020/may/12/will-coronavirus-lead-to-fairer-societies-thomas-piketty-explores-the-prospect).

Sridhar, D., *Preventable: How a Pandemic Changed the World and How to Stop the Next One* (London: Viking, 2022).

Staines, A. and Carey, D., '"Living with Covid" is empty sloganeering in need of a plan', *Irish Times*, 16 May 2022.

Stanford, P., 'Secular pilgrims: why ancient trails still pack a spiritual punch', *The Observer*, 28 March 2021 (https://www.theguardian.com/lifeandstyle/2021/mar/28/secular-pilgrims-why-ancient-trails-still-pack-a-spiritual-punch).

Stonor Saunders, F., *The Woman Who Shot Mussolini* (London: Faber and Faber, 2010).

Story, J.B., 'British Masters of Ophthalmology Series: 5.—Sir William Robert Wills Wilde (1815–1876)', *British Journal of Ophthalmology*, vol. 2 (1918), pp 63–71 (http://dx.doi.org/10.1136/bjo.2.2.nil1).

Sturgis, M., *Oscar: A Life* (London: Apollo/Head of Zeus, 2018).

Substance Abuse and Mental Health Services Administration, *Coping with Stress during Infectious Disease Outbreaks* (Rockville, MD: Substance Abuse and Mental Health Services Administration, 2014) (https://

store.samhsa.gov/product/Coping-with-Stress-During-Infectious-Disease-Outbreaks/sma14-4885).

Tait, A., 'Hope, high prices and long Covid', *The Observer*, 2 January 2022.

Taquet, M., Geddes, J.R., Husain, M., Luciano, S. and Harrison, P.J., '6-month neurological and psychiatric outcomes in 236 379 survivors of COVID-19: a retrospective cohort study using electronic health records', *Lancet Psychiatry*, vol. 8 (2021), pp 416–27 (https://doi.org/10.1016/S2215-0366(21)00084-5).

Taquet, M., Luciano, S., Geddes, J.R. and Harrison, P.J., 'Bidirectional associations between COVID-19 and psychiatric disorder: retrospective cohort studies of 62 354 COVID-19 cases in the USA', *Lancet Psychiatry*, vol. 8 (2021), pp 130–40 (https://doi.org/10.1016/S2215-0366(20)30462-4).

Taylor, S., 'I wrote the book on pandemic psychology. Post-Covid will take some getting used to', *The Guardian*, 24 February 2022 (https://www.theguardian.com/commentisfree/2022/feb/24/pandemic-psychology-end-covid-pandemic-normal).

Tóibín, C., *Mad, Bad, Dangerous to Know: The Fathers of Wilde, Yeats and Joyce* (London: Viking, 2018).

Vetter, P., Eckerle, I. and Kaiser, L., 'Covid-19: a puzzle with many missing pieces', *BMJ*, vol. 368 (2020), m627 (https://doi.org/10.1136/bmj.m627).

Vizheh, M., Qorbani, M., Arzaghi, S.M., Muhidin, S., Javanmard, Z. and Esmaeili, M., 'The mental health of healthcare workers in the COVID-19 pandemic: a systematic review', *Journal of Diabetes and Metabolic Disorders*, vol. 19 (2020), pp 1967–78 (https://doi.org/10.1007/s40200-020-00643-9).

Wallis, W., 'Experts fear mental illness crisis in Covid's wake', *Financial Times*, 27 February 2021.

Walsh, M., 'William Wilde: his contribution to otology', *Irish Journal of Medical Science*, vol. 185 (2016), pp 291–2 (https://doi.org/10.1007/s11845-016-1435-5).

Walshe, E., *The Diary of Mary Travers: A Novel* (Bantry: Somerville Press, 2014).

Waltner-Toews, D., *On Pandemics: Deadly Diseases from Bubonic Plague to Coronavirus* (Vancouver and Berkeley: Greystone Books, 2020).

Wang, C., Pan, R., Wan, X., Tan, Y., Xu, L., Ho, C.S. and Ho, R.C., 'Immediate psychological responses and associated factors during the initial stage of the 2019 coronavirus disease (COVID-19) epidemic among the general population in China', *International Journal of Environmental Research and Public Health*, vol. 17 (2020), p. 1729 (https://doi.org/10.3390/ijerph17051729).

Wang, G., Zhang, Y., Zhao, J., Zhang, J. and Jiang, F., 'Mitigate the effects of home confinement on children during the COVID-19 outbreak', *The Lancet*, vol. 395 (2020), pp 945–7 (https://doi.org/10.1016/S0140-6736(20)30547-X).

Wang, Q., Xu, R. and Volkow, N.D., 'Increased risk of COVID-19 infection and mortality in people with mental disorders: analysis from electronic health records in the United States', *World Psychiatry*, vol. 20 (2021), pp 124–30 (https://doi.org/10.1002/wps.20806).

Watts, J., 'Climate crisis: The virus gave us a chance to change. Are we taking it?', *The Guardian*, 30 December 2020 (https://www.theguardian.com/world/2020/dec/29/could-covid-lockdown-have-helped-save-the-planet).

Watts, M.T., 'Sir William Wilde 1815–1876: royal ophthalmologist extraordinary', *Journal of the Royal Society of Medicine*, vol. 83 (1990), pp 183–4 (https://doi.org/10.117 7/014107689008300318).

WHO Director-General, *WHO Director-General's Opening Remarks at the Media Briefing on COVID-19 (5 March 2020)* (Geneva: World Health Organization, 2020) (https://www.who.int/director-general/speeches/detail/who-director-general-s-opening-remarks-at-the-media-briefing-on-covid-19---5-march-2020).

Wilde, W.R., *Narrative of a Voyage to Madeira, Teneriffe, and Along the Shores of the Mediterranean, Including a Visit to Algiers, Egypt, Palestine, Tyre, Rhodes, Telmessus, Cyprus, and Greece, with Observations on the Present State and Prospects of Egypt and Palestine, and on the Climate, Natural History, Antiquities, etc. of the Countries Visited* (Dublin: William Curry, 1840).

Wilde, W.R., 'The editor's preface: The history of periodic medical literature in Ireland, including notices of the medical and philosophical societies of Dublin', *Dublin Quarterly Journal of Medical Science*, vol. 1 (1846), pp i–xlviii (https://doi.org/10.1007/BF02995525).

Wilde, W.R., 'Report upon the recent epidemic fever in Ireland', *Dublin Quarterly Journal of Medical Science*, vol. 7 (1849), pp 64–126 (https://doi.org/10.1007/BF02949643).

Wilde, W.R., 'Report upon the recent epidemic fever in Ireland', *Dublin Quarterly Journal of Medical Science*, vol. 7 (1849), pp 340–404 (https://doi.org/10.1007/BF02953227).

Wilde, W.R., 'Report upon the recent epidemic fever in Ireland', *Dublin Quarterly Journal of Medical Science*, vol. 8 (1849), pp 1–86 (https://doi.org/10.1007/BF03021167).

Wilde, W.R., 'Report upon the recent epidemic fever in Ireland', *Dublin Quarterly Journal of Medical Science*, vol. 8 (1849), pp 270–339 (https://doi.org/10.1007/BF02961754).

Wilde, W.R., *The Closing Years of Dean Swift's Life; With Remarks on Stella and on Some of His Writings Hitherto Unnoticed (Second Edition, Revised and Enlarged)* (Dublin: Hodges and Smith, 1849).

Wilde, W.R., *On the Physical, Moral, and Social Condition of the Deaf and Dumb* (London: John Churchill, 1854).

Wilde, W.R.W., *Ireland, Past and Present: The Land and the People: A Lecture* (Dublin: McGlashan and Gill, 1864).

Wilde, W.R.[W.], *Lough Corrib, its Shores and Islands: with Notices of Lough Mask* (Dublin: McGlashan and Gill, 1867).

Wilde, W.R., 'Memoir of Gabriel Beranger, and his labours in the cause of Irish art, literature, and antiquities, from 1760 to 1780, with illustrations', *Journal of the Royal*

Historical and Archaeological Association of Ireland, vol. 1 (1870), pp 33–64, 121–52, 236–60 (http://www.jstor.org/stable/25506575).

Wilde, W.R., *Memoir of Gabriel Beranger and His Labours in the Cause of Irish Art and Antiquities from 1760 to 1780* (Dublin: Gill and Son, 1880).

Williams, C., 'Heading for burnout?', *New Scientist*, vol. 249 (2021), pp 34–8.

Williams, R., 'Modern-day pilgrims beat a path to the Camino', *The Guardian*, 2 May 2011 (https://www.theguardian.com/travel/2011/may/02/camino-pilgrims-route).

Wilson, T.G., *Victorian Doctor: Being the Life of Sir William Wilde* (2nd edn) (London: Methuen, 1942).

Winter, G., 'Long Covid is "urgent" issue with "lingering psychological effects"', *Irish Times*, 11 January 2022.

Wong, S.Y.S., Zhang, D., Sit, R.W.S. *et al.*, 'Impact of COVID-19 on loneliness, mental health, and health service utilisation: a prospective cohort study of older adults with multimorbidity in primary care', *British Journal of General Practice*, vol. 70 (2020), e817–24 (https://doi.org/10.3399/bjgp20X713021).

Woolhouse, M., *The Year the World Went Mad: A Scientific Memoir* (Muir of Ord: Sandstone Press, 2022).

World Health Organization, *Mental Health and Psychosocial Considerations during the COVID-19 Outbreak* (Geneva: World Health Organization, 2020) (https://www.who.int/docs/default-source/coronaviruse/mental-health-considerations.pdf).

World Health Organization, *Report of the WHO–China Joint Mission on Coronavirus Disease 2019 (COVID-19)* (Geneva: World Health Organization, 2020) (https://www.who.int/docs/default-source/coronaviruse/who-china-joint-mission-on-covid-19-final-report.pdf).

World Health Organization, *COVID-19 Weekly Epidemiological Update (Data as Received by WHO from National Authorities, as of 14 March 2021, 10 am CET)* (Geneva: World Health Organization, 2021) (https://www.who.int/publications/m/item/weekly-epidemio-logical-update---16-march-2021).

Wright, L., *The Plague Year: America in the Time of Covid* (London: Allen Lane, 2021).

Zakaria, F., *Ten Lessons for a Post-Pandemic World* (London: Allen Lane, 2020).

Zarocostas, J., 'How to fight an infodemic', *The Lancet*, vol. 395 (2020), p. 676 (https://doi.org/10.1016/S0140-6736(20)30461-X).

ACKNOWLEDGEMENTS

I am very grateful to everyone who assisted me as I wrote this book. I deeply appreciate the support of my wife, Regina, and children, Eoin and Isabel. I am also very grateful to my parents, Mary and Desmond, my sisters, Sinéad and Niamh, and my nieces, Aoife and Aisling.

As ever, Trixie, Terry and the fish deserve special mention for bringing so much happiness into our lives.

I owe a long-standing debt of gratitude to my teachers at Scoil Chaitríona, Renmore, Galway; St Joseph's Patrician College, Nun's Island, Galway; and the School of Medicine at NUI Galway.

Many people helped me with this book. I am very grateful to Dr John Bruzzi, Dr Larkin Feeney, Professor Gautam Gulati, Mr Len Harrow, Mr Eoghan Marrow, Ms Harriet Wheelock (Keeper of Collections at the Royal College of Physicians of Ireland), the National Archives of Ireland, the Royal Irish Academy, the Royal Victoria Eye and Ear Hospital, Professor John Kelly and my other extraordinary work colleagues at Trinity College Dublin, Tallaght University Hospital and the Health Service Executive.

I am particularly grateful to Dr Aidan Collins for alerting me to, and giving me a beautiful copy of, Padraic Colum's *Moytura: A Play for Dancers* (Dublin: Dolmen Press, 1963). Thank you.

Finally, I am deeply grateful to my patients, their families and the many, many others who have helped and guided me along the way. Thank you, all.

PERMISSIONS

- Quotations from speeches and remarks of the President of Ireland are © President of Ireland.
- Information reused from MerrionStreet.ie is © MerrionStreet.ie.
- Some of the material in Chapter 1 is reprinted and adapted from B.D. Kelly, 'Plagues, pandemics and epidemics in Irish history prior to COVID-19 (coronavirus): what can we learn?', *Irish Journal of Psychological Medicine*, vol. 37 (2020), pp 269–74 (https://doi.org/10.1017/ipm.2020.25 [© The Author, 2020]). Published by Cambridge University Press on behalf of the *Irish Journal of Psychological Medicine*. Used with permission. Licence: https://creativecommons.org/licenses/by/4.0/.
- Some of the material in Chapter 1 is reprinted and adapted from B.D. Kelly, 'Vaccination is what makes this lockdown different to the last one', *The Echo Newspaper, Tallaght* 21 January 2021 (https://www.echo.

ie/vaccination-is-what-makes-this-lockdown-differ-ent-to-the-last-one/). It is adapted and reused by kind permission of *The Echo Newspaper, Tallaght.*

- Some of the material in Chapter 2 is reprinted and adapted from B.D. Kelly, 'We're all in an emotion-ally complex position—sharing our fears with others helps', *Irish Independent*, 24 March 2020 (https://www.independent.ie/opinion/comment/were-all-in-an-emo-tionally-complex-position-sharing-our-fears-with-oth-ers-helps-39070543.html). It is adapted and reused by kind permission of the *Irish Independent*.

- Some of the material in Chapter 2 previously appeared as a blogpost I wrote for *Psychology Today*: B.D. Kelly, 'Coping with coronavirus: if you want to be heard, listen (Blogpost)', *Psychology Today*, 25 March 2020 (https://www.psychologytoday.com/ie/blog/psychiatry-and-society/202003/coping-coronavirus-if-you-want-be-heard-listen [© Brendan Kelly]). It is reused and adapted here by permission.

- Some of the material in Chapter 3 previously appeared as a blogpost I wrote for *Psychology Today*: B.D. Kelly, 'COVID-19: real problems but no pandemic of mental illness (Blogpost)', *Psychology Today*, 17 November 2020 (https://www.psychologytoday.com/ie/blog/psychiatry-and-society/202011/covid-19-real-problems-no-pandemic-mental-illness [© Brendan Kelly]). It is reused and adapted here by permission.

- Some of the material in Chapter 4 previously appeared as a blogpost I wrote for *Psychology Today*: B.D. Kelly,

'Giving thanks in the time of Covid-19 (Blogpost)', *Psychology Today*, 25 April 2020 (https://www.psychologytoday.com/ie/blog/psychiatry-and-society/202004/giving-thanks-in-the-time-covid-19 [© Brendan Kelly]). It is reused and adapted here by permission.

- Some of the material in Chapter 5 previously appeared as a blogpost I wrote for *Psychology Today*: B.D. Kelly, 'What we've lost, how we'll recover (Blogpost)', *Psychology Today*, 20 May 2020 (https://www.psychologytoday.com/ie/blog/psychiatry-and-society/202005/what-weve-lost-how-well-recover [© Brendan Kelly]). It is reused and adapted here by permission.
- Material reproduced and adapted from the *Medical Independent* and *Update* is reproduced and adapted by kind permission of GreenCross Publishing.
- Extracts from *The Guardian* and *The Observer* are courtesy of *Guardian* News & Media Ltd.

I am very grateful to the editors, publishers, authors and copyright-holders who permitted reuse of material in this book. All reasonable efforts have been made to contact the copyright-holders for all material used. If any have been omitted, please contact the publisher. Many thanks.

ENDNOTES

INTRODUCTION

1   C. Murphy, 'Never forget—Covid inquiry must repair brain fog caused by ditching our values', *Sunday Independent*, 19 March 2023.

2   A. Doyle, 'Inquiry into response to Covid pandemic', *Irish Times*, 10 March 2023.

3   M. Cormican, 'Ireland's response to the SARS-CoV-2 pandemic. The Marianne Dashwood test', *ResearchGate*, October 2022 (https://www.researchgate.net/publication/365273684_ISCM_COVID_The_Marianne_Dashwood_Test_20102022_M_Cormican).

4   J. Horgan-Jones, H. O'Connell, *Pandemonium: Power, Politics and Ireland's Pandemic*. Dublin (Gill Books, 2022).

5   R. McEntegart, 'William Wilde and 1 Merrion Square', *Irish Journal of Medical Science*, vol. 185 (2016), pp 285–9 (https://doi.org/10.1007/s11845-016-1423-9).

6   P. Froggatt, 'Sir William Wilde, 1815–1876. A centenary appreciation: Wilde's place in medicine', *Proceedings of the Royal Irish Academy*, vol. 77C (1977), pp 261–78, at p. 262.

7   *Ibid.*, p. 266.

8   *Ibid.*, p. 270.

9   P. Froggatt, 'Sir William Wilde and the 1851 Census of Ireland', *Medical History*, vol. 9 (1965), 302–27 (https://doi.org/10.1017/s0025727300030970).

10 W. Donnelly and W.R. Wilde, *The Census of Ireland for the Year 1851, Part III: Report on the Status of Disease* (Dublin: Alexander Thom

and Sons, for Her Majesty's Stationery Office, 1854). (Wilde's census reports were co-signed by William Donnelly, Registrar-General and Chief Commissioner.)

11   W. Donnelly and W.R. Wilde, *The Census of Ireland for the Year 1851, Part V: Tables of Deaths. Volume I, Containing the Report, Tables of Pestilences, and Analysis of the Tables of Deaths* (Dublin: Alexander Thom and Sons, for Her Majesty's Stationery Office, 1856) (hereafter *Tables of Deaths*).

12   The second volume of Part V comes to 686 pages and presents more detailed tables of deaths along with additional statistical information; W. Donnelly and W.R. Wilde, *The Census of Ireland for the Year 1851, Part V: Tables of Deaths. Volume II, Containing the Tables and Index* (Dublin: Alexander Thom and Sons, for Her Majesty's Stationery Office, 1856).

13   *Tables of Deaths*, pp 43, 44 and 53.

14   *Ibid.*, p. 59.

15   *Ibid.*, p. 63.

16   *Ibid.*, pp 57 and 179.

17   *Ibid.*, p. 41.

18   *Ibid.*, pp 54, 59, 63 and 70.

19   W.R.W. Wilde, *Ireland, Past and Present: The Land and the People: A Lecture* (Dublin: McGlashan and Gill, 1864).

20   *Ibid.*, p. 2.

21   P. Froggatt, 'The demographic work of Sir William Wilde', *Irish Journal of Medical Science*, vol. 185 (2016), pp 293–5 (https://doi.org/10.1007/s11845-016-1436-4).

22   E. Butler, 'Graphic of the week: coffee consumption', *Irish Times*, 17 July 2021.

1. SPRING 2021: PLAGUE

1   A version of this passage appeared as: B.D. Kelly, 'Vaccination is what makes this lockdown different to the last one', *The Echo Newspaper, Tallaght*, 21 January 2021 (https://www.echo.ie/vaccination-is-what-makes-this-lockdown-different-to-the-last-one/). It

is adapted and reused by kind permission of *The Echo Newspaper, Tallaght*.

2   World Health Organization, *COVID-19 Weekly Epidemiological Update (Data as Received by WHO from National Authorities, as of 14 March 2021, 10 am CET)* (Geneva: World Health Organization, 2021) (https://www.who.int/publications/m/item/weekly-epidemiological-update---16-march-2021).

3   World Health Organization, *Report of the WHO–China Joint Mission on Coronavirus Disease 2019 (COVID-19)* (Geneva: World Health Organization, 2020) (https://www.who.int/docs/default-source/coronaviruse/who-china-joint-mission-on-covid-19-final-report.pdf). Some of the material in this section is reprinted and adapted from: B.D. Kelly, 'Plagues, pandemics and epidemics in Irish history prior to COVID-19 (coronavirus): what can we learn?', *Irish Journal of Psychological Medicine*, vol. 37 (2020), pp 269–74 (https://doi.org/10.1017/ipm.2020.25) (© The Author, 2020; published by Cambridge University Press on behalf of the *Irish Journal of Psychological Medicine*. Used with permission. Licence: https://creativecommons.org/licenses/by/4.0/).

4   '*The Guardian* view on tackling the new coronavirus: handle with care: editorial', *The Guardian*, 7 February 2020 (https://www.theguardian.com/commentisfree/2020/feb/07/the-guardian-view-on-tackling-the-new-coronavirus-handle-with-care [courtesy of *Guardian* News & Media Ltd]).

5   See https://www.rte.ie/news/2020/0320/1124382-covid-19-ireland-timeline/.

6   B.D. Kelly, 'Panic and hysteria will only weaken effort to halt virus', *Irish Times*, 2 March 2020 (https://www.irishtimes.com/opinion/panic-and-hysteria-will-undermine-efforts-to-contain-coronavirus-1.4189459).

7   M. Honigsbaum, *The Pandemic Century: One Hundred Years of Panic, Hysteria and Hubris* (London: C. Hurst, 2019).

8   C. Foley, *The Last Irish Plague: The Great Flu Epidemic in Ireland, 1918–19* (Dublin and Portland, OR: Irish Academic Press, 2011); M. Honigsbaum, 'The art of medicine. Spanish influenza redux: revisiting the mother of all pandemics', *The Lancet*, vol. 391 (2018), pp 2492–5 (https://doi.org/10.1016/S0140-6736(18)31360-6); I. Milne,

Stacking the Coffins: Influenza, War and Revolution in Ireland, 1918–19 (Manchester: Manchester University Press, 2018).

9   B.D. Kelly, *Coping with Coronavirus. How to Stay Calm and Protect Your Mental Health: A Psychological Toolkit* (Newbridge: Merrion Press, 2020), and 'Coronavirus: should we keep calm and carry on?', *The Guardian*, 9 March 2020.

10 W. Donnelly and W.R. Wilde, *The Census of Ireland for the Year 1851, Part V: Tables of Deaths. Volume I, Containing the Report, Tables of Pestilences, and Analysis of the Tables of Deaths* (Dublin: Alexander Thom and Sons, for Her Majesty's Stationery Office, 1856) (hereafter *Tables of Deaths*), p. 2.

11 *Ibid.*, p. 6.

12 *Ibid.*, p. 41.

13 *Ibid.*, p. 47.

14 *Ibid.*, p. 52.

15 *Ibid.*, p. 54.

16 *Ibid.*, p. 55.

17 *Ibid.*, p. 59.

18 See https://merrionstreet.ie/en/news-room/speeches/the_pandemic_one_year_on_-_speech_by_the_minister_for_finance_paschal_donohoe_t_d_to_the_economic_and_social_research_institute.167624.shortcut.html (© 2021 MerrionStreet.ie).

19 *Tables of Deaths*, p. 63.

20 *Ibid.*, p. 355.

21 J. Robins, *The Miasma: Epidemic and Panic in Nineteenth Century Ireland* (Dublin: Institute of Public Administration, 1995).

22 *Tables of Deaths*, p. 77.

23 *Ibid.*, p. 254.

24 B.D. Kelly, *Hearing Voices: The History of Psychiatry in Ireland* (Dublin: Irish Academic Press, 2016); D. Brennan, *Irish Insanity, 1800–2000* (London and New York: Routledge/Taylor and Francis, 2014).

25 Honigsbaum, 'The art of medicine'.

26 G. Beiner, P. Marsh and I. Milne, 'Greatest killer of the twentieth century: the Great Flu of 1918–19', *History Ireland*, vol. 17 (2) (2009), pp 40-3; Milne, *Stacking the Coffins*.

27 J. Robins, *Fools and Mad: A History of the Insane in Ireland* (Dublin: Institute of Public Administration, 1986).

28 G. Ferry, 'A woman's place. Dorothy Stopford Price and the control of tuberculosis in Ireland', *The Lancet*, vol. 393 (2019), p. 20 (https://doi.org/10.1016/S0140-6736(18)33171-4); A. Mac Lellan, *Dorothy Stopford Price: Rebel Doctor* (Dublin: Irish Academic Press, 2014).

29 K. Bielenberg, 'Be alert, but don't be alarmed!', *Irish Independent*, 7 March 2020.

30 R. Peckham, 'COVID-19 and the anti-lessons of history', *The Lancet*, vol. 395 (2020), pp 850–2 (https://doi.org/10.1016/S0140-6736(20)30468-2).

31 W. Hutton, 'Coronavirus won't end globalisation, but change it hugely for the better', *The Observer*, 8 March 2020 (https://www.theguardian.com/commentisfree/2020/mar/08/the-coronavirus-outbreak-shows-us-that-no-one-can-take-on-this-enemy-alone [courtesy of *Guardian* News & Media Ltd]).

32 T.G. Wilson, *Victorian Doctor: Being the Life of Sir William Wilde* (2nd edn) (London: Methuen, 1942).

33 W. Cullen, G. Gulati and B.D. Kelly, 'Mental health in the Covid-19 pandemic', *QJM*, vol. 113 (2020), pp 311–12 (https://doi.org/10.1093/qjmed/hcaa110); Milne, 'Learning from the past'.

34 C. Cookson, 'Beware fake news, do not panic buy and prepare for possible self-isolation', *Financial Times*, 7/8 March 2020; T. Harford, 'Falsehoods spread and mutate just like a virus', *Financial Times*, 7/8 March 2020.

35 Foley, *The Last Irish Plague*.

36 'COVID-19: fighting panic with information', *The Lancet*, vol. 395 (2020), p. 537 (https://doi.org/10.1016/S0140-6736(20)30379-2); J. Zarocostas, 'How to fight an infodemic', *The Lancet*, vol. 395 (2020), p. 676 (https://doi.org/10.1016/S0140-6736(20)30461-X).

37 'COVID-19: too little, too late?', *The Lancet*, vol. 395 (2020), p. 755 (https://doi.org/10.1016/S0140-6736(20)30522-5); M.S. Razai, K. Doerholt, S. Ladhani and P. Oakeshott, 'Coronavirus disease 2019 (covid-19): a guide for UK GPs', *BMJ*, vol. 368 (2020), m800 (https://doi.org/10.1136/bmj.m800).

38 Milne, *Stacking the Coffins*.

39 L. Duan and G. Zhu, 'Psychological interventions for people affected by the COVID-19 epidemic', *Lancet Psychiatry*, vol. 7 (2020), pp 300–2 (https://doi.org/10.1016/S2215-0366(20)30073-0).

40   J. Hellewell, S. Abbott, A. Gimma *et al.*, 'Feasibility of controlling
     COVID-19 outbreaks by isolation of cases and contacts', *Lancet
     Global Health*, vol. 8 (2020), e488–96 (https://doi.org/10.1016/
     S2214-109X(20)30074-7); S.K. Brooks, R.K. Webster, L.E. Smith,
     L. Woodland, S. Wessely, N. Greenberg and G.J. Rubin, 'The psy-
     chological impact of quarantine and how to reduce it: rapid review
     of the evidence', *The Lancet*, vol. 395 (2020), pp 912–20 (https://doi.
     org/10.1016/S0140-6736(20)30460-8).

41   G. Wang, Y. Zhang, J. Zhao, J. Zhang and F. Jiang, 'Mitigate the
     effects of home confinement on children during the COVID-19 out-
     break', *The Lancet*, vol. 395 (2020), pp 945–7 (https://doi.org/10.1016/
     S0140-6736(20)30547-X).

42   S. Jenkins, 'Was I wrong? Even scientists still don't agree on
     Covid-19', *The Guardian*, 3 April 2020 (https://www.theguardian.
     com/commentisfree/2020/apr/02/wrong-coronavirus-world-
     scientists-optimism-experts [courtesy of *Guardian* News &
     Media Ltd]).

43   P. Vetter, I. Eckerle and L. Kaiser, 'Covid-19: a puzzle with many
     missing pieces', *BMJ*, vol. 368 (2020), m627 (https://doi.org/10.1136/
     bmj.m627); T. Ord, 'The importance of worst-case thinking', *The
     Guardian*, 6 March 2020; S. Jenkins, 'Let them wash your hands, but
     not your brain', *The Guardian,* 7 March 2020; H. Mance, 'A shock to
     the system', *Financial Times*, 7/8 March 2020; J. Naughton, 'How a
     global health crisis turns into a state-run surveillance opportunity',
     The Observer, 8 March 2020; Y.N. Harari, 'The world after coronavi-
     rus', *Financial Times*, 21/22 March 2020.

44   Substance Abuse and Mental Health Services Administration, *Coping
     with Stress during Infectious Disease Outbreaks* (Rockville, MD:
     Substance Abuse and Mental Health Services Administration, 2014)
     (https://store.samhsa.gov/product/Coping-with-Stress-During-
     Infectious-Disease-Outbreaks/sma14-4885); P. Chödrön, *When Things
     Fall Apart: Heart Advice for Difficult Times* (Boulder, CO: Shambala
     Publications, 2016); Kelly, *Coping with Coronavirus*; World Health
     Organization, *Mental Health and Psychosocial Considerations during
     the COVID-19 Outbreak* (Geneva: World Health Organization,
     2020) (https://www.who.int/docs/default-source/coronaviruse/
     mental-health-considerations.pdf); Centers for Disease Control and

Prevention, *Manage Anxiety and Stress* (Atlanta, GA: Centers for Disease Control and Prevention, 2020).

45 Q. Wang, R. Xu and N.D. Volkow, 'Increased risk of COVID-19 infection and mortality in people with mental disorders: analysis from electronic health records in the United States', *World Psychiatry*, vol. 20 (2021), pp 124–30 (https://doi.org/10.1002/wps.20806).

46 M. Rodgers, J. Dalton, M. Harden, A. Street, G. Parker and A. Eastwood, 'Integrated care to address the physical health needs of people with severe mental illness: a mapping review of the recent evidence on barriers, facilitators and evaluations', *International Journal of Integrated Care*, vol. 18 (2018), p. 9 (https://doi.org/10.5334/ijic.2605).

47 WHO Director-General, *WHO Director-General's Opening Remarks at the Media Briefing on COVID-19 (5 March 2020)* (Geneva: World Health Organization, 2020) (https://www.who.int/director-general/speeches/detail/who-director-general-s-opening-remarks-at-the-media-briefing-on-covid-19---5-march-2020).

48 B.D. Kelly, 'The spread of disease is always political but then so is the cure', *Financial Times*, 2/3 May 2020.

49 See https://president.ie/en/media-library/speeches/address-to-the-aepi-webconference-responding-to-covid-19-the-situation-in-africa [© 2020 President of Ireland]).

50 See https://president.ie/en/diary/details/president-hosts-a-reception-commemorating-the-great-flu-epidemic-of-1918-1919/speeches [© 2019 President of Ireland]).

51 W.R. Wilde, *Lough Corrib, its Shores and Islands: with Notices of Lough Mask* (Dublin: McGlashan and Gill, 1867), p. 280.

52 *Ibid.*, p. 284.

53 *Ibid.*, p. 27.

54 *Ibid.*, p. 218.

55 *Tables of Deaths*, p. 355.

56 See https://merrionstreet.ie/en/news-room/news/statement_of_an_taoiseach_leo_varadkar_t_d_update_on_covid-19_emergency_.html [© 2020 MerrionStreet.ie]).

57 T. Jones, 'The rebirth of humanity', *The Observer*, 12 April 2020 (https://www.theguardian.com/world/2020/apr/12/after-coronavirus-the-penny-has-dropped-that-wellbeing-isnt-individual-but-social [courtesy of *Guardian* News & Media Ltd]).

58 *Tables of Deaths*, pp 39–40. See also B.D. Kelly, 'Pandemics and the lessons of history', *Irish Times*, 14 August 2021 (https://www.irishtimes.com/opinion/letters/pandemics-and-the-lessons-of-history-1.4646534).

2. SUMMER 2021: COPING

1   See https://merrionstreet.ie/en/news-room/releases/statement_from_the_national_public_health_emergency_team.html.

2   R. Horton, *The Covid-19 Catastrophe: What's Gone Wrong and How to Stop it Happening Again* (Cambridge: Polity Press, 2020).

3   W.R. Wilde, *Narrative of a Voyage to Madeira, Teneriffe, and Along the Shores of the Mediterranean, Including a Visit to Algiers, Egypt, Palestine, Tyre, Rhodes, Telmessus, Cyprus, and Greece, with Observations on the Present State and Prospects of Egypt and Palestine, and on the Climate, Natural History, Antiquities, etc. of the Countries Visited* (Dublin: William Curry, 1840) (hereafter *Narrative of a Voyage*), pp v–vi.

4   *Ibid.*, vol. 1, p. 1.

5   *Ibid.*, vol. 1, p. 8.

6   *Ibid.*, vol. 1, pp 8–9.

7   *Ibid.*, vol. 1, p. 82.

8   *Ibid.*, vol. 1, p. 111.

9   *Ibid.*, vol. 1, pp 130–1.

10 *Ibid.*, vol. 1, pp 132–3.

11 Some of this passage is reprinted and adapted from B.D. Kelly, 'We're all in an emotionally complex position—sharing our fears with others helps', *Irish Independent*, 24 March 2020 (https://www.independent.ie/opinion/comment/were-all-in-an-emotionally-complex-position-sharing-our-fears-with-others-helps-39070543.html). It is adapted and reused by kind permission of the *Irish Independent*.

12 *Narrative of a Voyage,* vol. 1, pp 169–70.

13 T.G. Wilson, *Victorian Doctor: Being the Life of Sir William Wilde* (New York: L.B. Fischer, 1946), p. 43.

14 *Narrative of a Voyage,* vol. 1, p. 185.

15 *Ibid.*, vol. 1, pp 187–8.

16   *Ibid.*, vol. 1, pp 188–9.

17   *Ibid.*, vol. 1, pp 219–20.

18   *Ibid.*, vol. 1, pp 234–5.

19   *Ibid.*, vol. 1, pp 246–7.

20   R.J. Defalque and A.J. Wright, 'Travers vs. Wilde and other: chloroform acquitted', *Bulletin of Anesthesia History*, vol. 23 (1) (2005), pp 4–7 (https://doi.org/10.1016/s1522-8649(05)50045-3).

21   Part of this passage previously appeared as a blogpost I wrote for *Psychology Today*: B.D. Kelly, 'Coping with coronavirus: if you want to be heard, listen (Blogpost)', *Psychology Today*, 25 March 2020 (https://www.psychologytoday.com/ie/blog/psychiatry-and-society/202003/coping-coronavirus-if-you-want-be-heard-listen [© Brendan Kelly]). It is reused and adapted here by permission.

22   B.D. Kelly, *Coping with Coronavirus: How to Stay Calm and Protect Your Mental Health: A Psychological Toolkit* (Dublin: Merrion Press, 2020).

23   W.R. Wilde, *Lough Corrib, its Shores and Islands: with Notices of Lough Mask* (Dublin: McGlashan and Gill, 1867).

24   H. Speakman, *Here's Ireland* (London: Arrowsmith, 1926), p. 142.

25   *Narrative of a Voyage,* vol. 1, p. 312.

26   *Ibid.*, vol. 1, p. 329.

27   *Ibid.*, vol. 1, p. 322.

28   *Ibid.*, vol. 2, pp 45–6.

29   *Ibid.*, vol. 2, p. 466.

30   T. de Vere White, *The Parents of Oscar Wilde: Sir William and Lady Wilde* (London: Hodder and Stoughton, 1967), p. 64.

31   See https://merrionstreet.ie/en/news-room/releases/speech_by_the_taoiseach_michel_martin_-_covid-19_reframing_the_challenge_continuing_our_recovery_reconnecting.html).

32   L. Wright, *The Plague Year: America in the Time of Covid* (London: Allen Lane, 2021).

3. AUTUMN 2021: NOT COPING

1   B. Quinn, 'Covid-19 deaths among the fully vaccinated represent just 1.2% of total in England', *The Guardian*, 14 September 2021 (https://

www.theguardian.com/world/2021/sep/13/fully-vaccinated-people-account-for-12-of-englands-covid-19-deaths [courtesy of *Guardian* News & Media Ltd]).

2   See https://www.rte.ie/news/coronavirus/2021/0921/1247997-us-coronavirus-world/.

3   'Vaccinating the world', *The Economist*, 15 May 2021.

4   B.D. Kelly, 'Coronavirus disease: challenges for psychiatry', *British Journal of Psychiatry*, vol. 217 (2020), pp 352–3 (https://doi.org/10.1192/bjp.2020.86); M.M. Hossain, S. Tasnim, A. Sultana *et al.*, 'Epidemiology of mental health problems in COVID-19: a review', *F1000Research*, vol. 9 (2020), p. 636 (https://doi.org/10.12688/f1000research.24457.1).

5   B.D. Kelly, 'Impact of Covid-19 on mental health in Ireland: evidence to date', *Irish Medical Journal*, vol. 113 (2020), pp 214–17 (http://imj.ie/impact-of-covid-19-on-mental-health-in-ireland-evidence-to-date/).

6   C. Wang, R. Pan, X. Wan, Y. Tan, L. Xu, C.S. Ho and R.C. Ho, 'Immediate psychological responses and associated factors during the initial stage of the 2019 coronavirus disease (COVID-19) epidemic among the general population in China', *International Journal of Environmental Research and Public Health*, vol. 17 (2020), p. 1729 (https://doi.org/10.3390/ijerph17051729).

7   L. García-Álvarez, L. de la Fuente-Tomás, M.P. García-Portilla *et al.*, 'Early psychological impact of the 2019 coronavirus disease (COVID-19) pandemic and lockdown in a large Spanish sample', *Journal of Global Health*, vol. 10 (2020), 020505 (https://doi.org/10.7189/jogh.10.020505).

8   T. Burke, A. Berry, L.K. Taylor *et al.*, 'Increased psychological distress during COVID-19 and quarantine in Ireland: a national survey', *Journal of Clinical Medicine*, vol. 9 (2020), E3481 (https://doi.org/10.3390/jcm9113481).

9   P. Hyland, F. Vallières, M. Shevlin, J. Murphy, O. McBride, T. Karatzias and R. Bentall, *COVID-19 mental health survey by Maynooth University and Trinity College finds high rates of anxiety* (Maynooth: Maynooth University, 2020) (https://www.maynoothuniversity.ie/news-events/covid-19-mental-health-survey-maynooth-university-and-trinity-college-finds-high-rates-anxiety).

10   Part of this passage is an adaptation of a blogpost I wrote for
      Psychology Today: B.D. Kelly, 'COVID-19: real problems but no pan-
      demic of mental illness (Blogpost)', *Psychology Today*, 17 November
      2020 (https://www.psychologytoday.com/ie/blog/psychiatry-and-so-
      ciety/202011/covid-19-real-problems-no-pandemic-mental-illness [©
      Brendan Kelly]). It is reused and adapted here by permission. See also
      B.D. Kelly, 'Covid-19 and mental health', *Irish Times*, 26 November
      2020.

11   College of Psychiatrists of Ireland, *COVID-19 Impact on Secondary
      Mental Healthcare Services in Ireland* (Dublin: College of
      Psychiatrists of Ireland, 2020) (https://www.irishpsychiatry.ie/
      external-affairs-policy/college-papers-submissions-publications/
      positions-policies-perspective-papers/covid-19-impact-on-second-
      ary-mental-healthcare-services-in-ireland/).

12   College of Psychiatrists of Ireland, 'Press Statement', 17 June 2020
      (https://www.irishpsychiatry.ie/external-affairs-policy/college-pa-
      pers-submissions-publications/positions-policies-perspective-papers/
      covid-19-impact-on-secondary-mental-healthcare-services-in-ire-
      land/).

13   F. McNicholas and K. Moore, 'Covid-19, child and adolescent
      mental health services (CAMHS) and crises', *Irish Medical Journal*,
      vol. 115 (2022), p. 522 (http://imj.ie/covid-19-child-adolescent-men-
      tal-health-services-camhs-and-crises/).

14   S.K. Brooks, R.K. Webster, L.E. Smith, L. Woodland, S. Wessely, N.
      Greenberg and G.J. Rubin, 'The psychological impact of quarantine
      and how to reduce it: rapid review of the evidence', *The Lancet*, vol.
      395 (2020), pp 912–20 (https://doi.org/10.1016/S0140-6736(20)30460-
      8).

15   S. Bracken, 'Hospital figures for self-harm fall 25%', *Irish Times*, 12
      September 2020.

16   College of Psychiatrists of Ireland, 'Press Statement', 17 June 2020.

17   S.Y.S. Wong, D. Zhang, R.W.S. Sit *et al.*, 'Impact of COVID-19 on
      loneliness, mental health, and health service utilisation: a prospective
      cohort study of older adults with multimorbidity in primary care',
      British Journal of General Practice, vol. 70 (2020), e817–24 (https://
      doi.org/10.3399/bjgp20X713021).

18   I.W.C. Mak, P.M. Chu, P.C. Pan, M.G.C. Yiu and V.L. Chan, 'Long-term psychiatric morbidities among SARS survivors', *General Hospital Psychiatry*, vol. 31 (2009), pp 318–26 (https://doi.org/10.1016/j.gen-hosppsych.2009.03.001).

19   Hossain *et al.*, 'Epidemiology of mental health problems in COVID-19: a review'.

20   Q. Guo, Y. Zheng, J. Shi *et al.*, 'Immediate psychological distress in quarantined patients with COVID-19 and its association with peripheral inflammation: a mixed-method study', *Brain, Behavior, and Immunity*, vol. 88 (2020), pp 17–27 (https://doi.org/10.1016/j.bbi.2020.05.038).

21   M. Taquet, S. Luciano, J.R. Geddes and P.J. Harrison, 'Bidirectional associations between COVID-19 and psychiatric disorder: retrospective cohort studies of 62354 COVID-19 cases in the USA', *Lancet Psychiatry*, vol. 8 (2021), pp 130–40 (https://doi.org/10.1016/S2215-0366(20)30462-4).

22   G. Douaud, S. Lee, F. Alfaro-Almagro *et al.*, 'SARS-CoV-2 is associated with changes in brain structure in UK Biobank', *Nature*, vol. 604 (2022), pp 697–707 (https://doi.org/10.1038/s41586-022-04569-5).

23   Brooks *et al.*, 'The psychological impact of quarantine and how to reduce it'.

24   K. O'Connor, M. Wrigley, R. Jennings, M. Hill and A. Niazi, 'Mental health impacts of COVID-19 in Ireland and the need for a secondary care mental health service response', *Irish Journal of Psychological Medicine*, vol. 38 (2021), pp 99–107 (https://doi.org/10.1017/ipm.2020.64).

25   College of Psychiatrists of Ireland, *COVID-19 Impact on Secondary Mental Healthcare Services in Ireland*.

26   A. McIntyre, K. Tong, E. McMahon and A.M. Doherty, 'COVID-19 and its effect on emergency presentations to a tertiary hospital with self-harm in Ireland', *Irish Journal of Psychological Medicine*, vol. 38 (2021), pp 116–22 (https://doi.org/10.1017/ipm.2020.116).

27   B.D. Kelly, 'Are we finally making progress with suicide and self-harm? An overview of the history, epidemiology and evidence for prevention', *Irish Journal of Psychological Medicine*, vol. 35 (2018), pp 95–101 (https://doi.org/10.1017/ipm.2017.51).

28   M. Naghavi on behalf of the Global Burden of Disease Self-Harm
Collaborators, 'Global, regional, and national burden of suicide
mortality 1990 to 2016: systematic analysis for the Global Burden
of Disease Study 2016', *BMJ*, vol. 364 (2019), p. 194 (https://doi.
org/10.1136/bmj.194).

29   HSE National Office for Suicide Prevention, *Annual Report 2019*
(Dublin: Health Service Executive, 2020) (https://www.hse.ie/eng/
services/list/4/mental-health-services/connecting-for-life/publica-
tions/nosp-annual-report-2019.pdf); B.D. Kelly, 'The effects of the
Covid-19 pandemic on suicide and self-harm', *Update: Psychiatry and
Neurology*, vol. 7 (2021), pp 20–1.

30   F.B. Ahmad and R.N. Anderson, 'The leading causes of death in
the US for 2020', *JAMA*, vol. 325 (2021), pp 1829–30 (https://doi.
org/10.1001/jama.2021.5469).

31   V. Efstathiou, M.-I. Stefanou, N. Siafakas *et al.*, 'Suicidality and
COVID-19: suicidal ideation, suicidal behaviors and completed
suicides amidst the COVID-19 pandemic (review)', *Experimental and
Therapeutic Medicine*, vol. 23 (2022), p. 107 (https://doi.org/10.3892/
etm.2021.11030). For media analysis, see S. Corrigan, 'No evidence
of suicide spike', *Connacht Tribune*, 12 February 2021; K. Holland,
'Suicides have not increased in past year, figures show', *Irish Times*,
2 March 2021; M. Joyce, E. Arensman and E. Griffin, 'No visible
increase in suicides in pandemic', *Irish Examiner*, 30 April 2021.

32   Healthy Ireland, Department of Health, Health Service Executive and
National Office for Suicide Prevention, *Connecting for Life: Ireland's
National Strategy to Reduce Suicide, 2015–2020* (Dublin: Department
of Health, 2015) (http://health.gov.ie/wp-content/uploads/2015/06/
Connecting-for-Life_LR.pdf).

33   Kelly, 'Are we finally making progress with suicide and self-harm?'.

34   W.R. Wilde, *The Closing Years of Dean Swift's Life; With Remarks on
Stella and on Some of His Writings Hitherto Unnoticed (Second Edition,
Revised and Enlarged)* (Dublin: Hodges and Smith, 1849).

35   B.D. Kelly, *Hearing Voices: The History of Psychiatry in Ireland*
(Dublin: Irish Academic Press, 2016), p. 22.

36   E. Malcolm, *Swift's Hospital: A History of St Patrick's Hospital, Dublin,
1746–1989* (Dublin: Gill and Macmillan, 1989), p. 6. See also T.P.C.
Kirkpatrick, *A Note on the History of the Care of the Insane in Ireland*

up to the End of the Nineteenth Century (Dublin: University Press, Ponsonby and Gibbs, 1931), p. 15; T.P.C. Kirkpatrick, 'Obituary: Richard Robert Leeper', *Journal of Mental Science*, vol. 88 (1942), pp 480–1 (https://doi.org/10.1192/bjp.88.372.480).

37 Malcolm, *Swift's Hospital*, pp 1–3.

38 Wilde, *The Closing Years of Dean Swift's Life*, p. 78.

39 *Ibid.*, p. 27.

40 *Ibid.*, p. 64.

41 *Ibid.*, p. 65.

42 *Ibid.*, p. 67.

43 T.H. Bewley, 'The health of Jonathan Swift', *Journal of the Royal Society of Medicine*, vol. 91 (1998), pp 602–5 (https://doi.org/10.1177/014107689809101118); T. Bewley, 'Swift's pocky quean', *Journal of the Royal Society of Medicine*, vol. 92 (1999), p. 216 (https://doi.org/10.1177/014107689909200427); C. Arnold, *Bedlam: London and its Mad* (London: Simon and Schuster/Pocket Books, 2009), p. 100; B.D. Kelly, *Custody, Care and Criminality: Forensic Psychiatry and Law in 19th Century Ireland* (Dublin: History Press Ireland, 2014), p. 158; L. O'Brien, 'The magic wisp: a history of the mentally ill in Ireland', *Bulletin of the Menninger Clinic*, vol. 31 (1967), pp 79–95, at p. 83.

44 A.W. Clare, 'Swift, mental illness and St Patrick's Hospital', *Irish Journal of Psychological Medicine*, vol. 15 (1998), pp 100–4, at p. 103 (https://doi.org/10.1017/S0790966700003797).

45 W.R. Brain, 'The illness of Dean Swift', *Irish Journal of Medical Science*, vol. 320–1 (1952), pp 337–45 (https://doi.org/10.1007/BF02956890).

46 Wilde, *The Closing Years of Dean Swift's Life*, p. 55.

47 *Ibid.*, p. 72.

48 *Ibid.*, p. 79.

49 *Ibid.*, p. 86.

50 P. Gilligan, 'Chief Executive's Foreword', in *St Patrick's Mental Health Services Annual Report and Financial Statements 2020* (Dublin: St Patrick's Mental Health Services, 2021), pp 4–5 (https://www.stpatricks.ie/media-centre/news/2021/july/annualandoutcomesreport2020).

51 See https://www.stpatricks.ie/media-centre/news/2021/august/mental-health-stigma-survey-2021.

52 C. McCarrick, A. Gribben and D. Lyons, 'To have and to hold: repercussions of lockdown in psychiatry', *Hospital Doctor of Ireland*, vol. 27 (2021), pp 25–8.

53 M. Vizheh, M. Qorbani, S.M. Arzaghi, S. Muhidin, Z. Javanmard and M. Esmaeili, 'The mental health of healthcare workers in the COVID-19 pandemic: a systematic review', *Journal of Diabetes and Metabolic Disorders*, vol. 19 (2020), pp 1967–78 (https://doi.org/10.1007/s40200-020-00643-9).

54 J. Coto, A. Restrepo, I. Cejas and S. Prentiss, 'The impact of COVID-19 on allied health professions', *PLoS ONE*, vol. 15 (2020), e0241328 (https://doi.org/10.1371/journal.pone.0241328).

55 S. O'Hagan, ' The psychological cost of Covid-19', *The Observer*, 7 June 2020 (https://www.theguardian.com/world/2020/jun/07/health-experts-on-the-psychological-cost-of-covid-19 [courtesy of *Guardian* News & Media Ltd]).

56 W. Cullen, G. Gulati and B.D. Kelly, 'Mental health in the Covid-19 pandemic', *QJM*, vol. 113 (2020), pp 311–12 (https://doi.org/10.1093/qjmed/hcaa110); C. Williams, 'Heading for burnout?', *New Scientist*, vol. 249 (2021), pp 34–8; P. Harrold, 'Burned out GPs boosted from giving first round of jabs', *Irish Times*, 23 March 2021; I. Kelly, 'Many lessons in public health learned this year', *Irish Examiner*, 19 April 2021; V. Hitzeroth and I. Lavelle, 'Looking after the medics during the pandemic', *Irish Medical Times*, vol. 55 (2021), p. 16.

57 J. Lai, S. Ma, Y. Wang *et al.*, 'Factors associated with mental health outcomes among health care workers exposed to coronavirus disease 2019', *JAMA Network Open*, vol. 3 (2020), e203976 (https://doi.org/10.1001/jamanetworkopen.2020.3976).

58 G. Gulati, B.D. Kelly, C.P. Dunne and L. Glynn, 'Rise in violence in general practice settings during the COVID-19 pandemic: implications for prevention', *Family Practice*, vol. 38 (2021), pp 696–8 (https://doi.org/10.1093/fampra/cmab060).

59 S.J. Foley, A. O'Loughlin and J. Creedon, 'Early experiences of radiographers in Ireland during the COVID-19 crisis', *Insights into Imaging*, vol. 11 (2020), p. 104 (https://doi.org/10.1186/s13244-020-00910-6).

60 College of Psychiatrists of Ireland, *COVID-19 Impact on Secondary Mental Healthcare Services in Ireland*.

61 Kelly, 'Impact of Covid-19 on mental health in Ireland: evidence to date'.

62 B. Gavin, J. Hayden, D. Adamis and F. McNicholas, 'Caring for the psychological well-being of healthcare professionals in the Covid-19 pandemic crisis', *Irish Medical Journal*, vol. 113 (2020), pp 51–3 (http://imj.ie/caring-for-the-psychological-well-being-of-front-line-workers-during-covid-19/).

63 E. Minihan, B. Gavin, B.D. Kelly and F. McNicholas, 'COVID-19, mental health and psychological first aid', *Irish Journal of Psychological Medicine*, vol. 37 (2020), pp 259–63 (https://doi.org/10.1017/ipm.2020.41).

64 College of Psychiatrists of Ireland, 'Press Statement', 17 June 2020.

65 B. Levin, 'The questions machines cannot answer', *The Times*, 3 October 1978.

66 T.G. Wilson, *Victorian Doctor: Being the Life of Sir William Wilde* (2nd edn) (London: Methuen, 1942), pp 95, 120.

67 Part of this passage appeared as B.D. Kelly, 'Kay proves again why he is publishing's gain and medicine's loss', *Medical Independent*, 16 December 2022 (https://www.medicalindependent.ie/life/book-review/kay-proves-again-why-he-is-publishings-gain-and-medicines-loss/). It is reproduced and adapted by kind permission of GreenCross Publishing.

68 See https://www.rte.ie/news/2022/0528/1301698-irish-medical-organisation/.

69 G. Gulati and B.D. Kelly, 'Physician suicide and the COVID-19 pandemic', *Occupational Medicine*, vol. 70 (2020), p. 514 (https://doi.org/10.1093/occmed/kqaa104).

70 'The fourth wave', *The Economist*, 27 November 2021.

71 M. Houston, 'Do we need to reassess our confidence in Covid vaccine?', *Irish Times*, 2 November 2021.

72 See, for example, M. Paul, 'Government didn't do enough to stop this surge', *Irish Times*, 19 November 2021.

73 R. Chambers, *A State of Emergency: The Story of Ireland's Covid Crisis* (Dublin: HarperCollinsIreland, 2021).

74 Fianna Fáil South County Dublin Constituency Convention, Glenalbyn Sports Centre, Stillorgan, Dublin (5 February 1978).

75 A.W. Clare, *A Study of Psychiatric Illness in an Immigrant Irish Population* (MPhil. (Psychiatry) thesis, University of London, 1972).

76 B.D. Kelly and M. Houston, *Psychiatrist in the Chair: The Official Biography of Anthony Clare* (Dublin: Merrion Press, 2020), pp 41–4.

77 Kelly, *Hearing Voices*, pp 206–9.

78 B.D. Kelly, 'What does being Irish mean to me, in M.-C. Logue (ed.), *Being Irish: 101 Views on Irish Identity Today* (Dublin: The Liffey Press, 2021), pp 128–30.

79 J. Henley and P. Oltermann, 'Why is Europe returning to the dark days of Covid?', *The Observer*, 14 November 2021 (https://www.theguardian.com/world/2021/nov/13/why-is-europe-returning-to-the-dark-days-of-covid [courtesy of *Guardian* News & Media Ltd]).

80 K. Mills, 'Emergence of new variant adds to urgency of booster campaign', *Irish Times*, 27 November 2021.

81 Q.Q. Wang, R. Xu and N.D. Volkow, 'Increased risk of COVID-19 infection and mortality in people with mental disorders: analysis from electronic health records in the United States', *World Psychiatry*, vol. 20 (2021), pp 124–30 (https://doi.org/10.1002/wps.20806). See also M. Houston, 'Covid-19 and its effects on our mental health', *Irish Times*, 15 June 2021.

82 J. Robins, *Fools and Mad: A History of the Insane in Ireland* (Dublin: Institute of Public Administration, 1986), p. 180.

83 B.D. Kelly, 'Covid-19 and mental illness', *Irish Times*, 27 April 2020.

84 S. Finnerty, *Physical Health of People with Severe Mental Illness* (Dublin: Mental Health Commission, 2019), p. 5 (https://www.mhcirl.ie/publications/physical-health-people-severe-mental-illness).

85 M. De Hert, V. Mazereel, J. Detraux and K. Van Assche, 'Prioritizing COVID-19 vaccination for people with severe mental illness', *World Psychiatry*, vol. 20 (2021), pp 54–5 (https://doi.org/10.1002/wps.20826).

86 C. Henry, 'Covid-19 is not just affecting our bodies—it's also getting us down', *Irish Medical Times*, 10 November 2021.

87 G. Gulati and B.D. Kelly, 'Domestic violence against women and the Covid-19 pandemic: what is the role of psychiatry?', *International Journal of Law and Psychiatry*, vol. 71 (2020), p. 101594 (https://doi.org/10.1016/j.ijlp.2020.101594); D. Lynch, 'Drinking patterns in the pandemic', *Medical Independent*, 27 January 2022.

88   G. Gulati, C.P. Dunne and B.D. Kelly, 'Do COVID-19
      responses imperil the human rights of people with disabilities?',
      Health and Human Rights Journal, 3 June 2020 (https://www.
      hhrjournal.org/2020/06/do-covid-19-responses-imperil-the-hu-
      man-rights-of-people-with-disabilities/).

89   D. Fujiwara, P. Dolan, R. Lawton, F. Behzadnejad, A. Lagarde,
      C. Maxwell and S. Peytrignet, *The Wellbeing Costs of COVID-19
      in the UK: An Independent Research Report by Simetrica-Jacobs and
      the London School of Economics and Political Science* (London:
      Simetrica-Jacobs and the London School of Economics and Political
      Science, 2020), p. 3 (https://www.lse.ac.uk/News/Latest-news-from-
      LSE/2020/e-May-20/Wellbeing-and-COVID-19).

90   D. Adeluwoye, 'Mental health problems soar for young people during
      lockdown', *The Observer*, 30 August 2020; W. Wallis, 'Experts fear
      mental illness crisis in Covid's wake', *Financial Times*, 27 February
      2021; I. Sample, 'Covid's impact on mental health will last years, royal
      college warns', *The Guardian*, 28 December 2020.

91   R. Bentall, 'Has the pandemic really caused a "tsunami" of mental
      health problems?', *The Guardian*, 9 February 2021.

92   See https://www.who.int/docs/default-source/coronaviruse/men-
      tal-health-considerations.pdf; https://www.cdc.gov/mentalhealth/
      stress-coping/cope-with-stress/index.html; https://www2.hse.ie/
      wellbeing/mental-health/covid-19/minding-your-mental-health-dur-
      ing-the-coronavirus-outbreak.html.

93   B.D. Kelly, 'Coping with coronavirus: how to stay calm and protect
      your mental health (Blogpost)', *Lust for Life*, 19 January 2021 (https://
      www.alustforlife.com/tools/coping-with-coronavirus-how-to-stay-
      calm-and-protect-your-mental-health).

94   B.D. Kelly, 'Mind your mental health during this most psychologically
      difficult phase of the pandemic', *Irish Independent*, 25 August 2020.

95   B.D. Kelly, 'How to protect your mental health during the Covid-19
      pandemic', *Update: Psychiatry and Neurology*, vol. 7 (2021), pp 26–7.

96   E. Shafak, *How to Stay Sane in an Age of Division* (London: Profile
      Books and Wellcome Collection, 2020), p. 81.

97   See https://president.ie/en/media-library/speeches/reflecting-on-cov-
      id19-solidarity-care-compassion-and-kindness (© 2020 President of
      Ireland).

4. WINTER 2021: WORKING

1   C. Tóibín, *Mad, Bad, Dangerous to Know: The Fathers of Wilde, Yeats and Joyce* (London: Viking, 2018), pp 23–76.

2   R. Foster, 'Sins of the fathers', *The Spectator*, 15 December 2018.

3   J.B. Story, 'British Masters of Ophthalmology Series: 5.—Sir William Robert Wills Wilde (1815–1876)', *British Journal of Ophthalmology*, vol. 2 (1918), pp 63–71 (http://dx.doi.org/10.1136/bjo.2.2.nil1).

4   W.R. Wilde, *Narrative of a Voyage to Madeira, Teneriffe, and Along the Shores of the Mediterranean, Including a Visit to Algiers, Egypt, Palestine, Tyre, Rhodes, Telmessus, Cyprus, and Greece, with Observations on the Present State and Prospects of Egypt and Palestine, and on the Climate, Natural History, Antiquities, etc. of the Countries Visited* (Dublin: William Curry, 1840), vol. 1, pp 246–7; G. Crookes, *Dublin's Eye and Ear: The Making of a Monument* (Dublin: Town House, 1993), pp 9–10; R.J. Defalque and A.J. Wright, 'Travers vs. Wilde and other: chloroform acquitted', *Bulletin of Anesthesia History*, vol. 23 (4) (2005), pp 1, 4–7 (https://doi.org/10.1016/s1522-8649(05)50045-3).

5   M. Ivanišević, 'Albrecht von Graefe's ophthalmic educational visit to William Wilde in Dublin in 1851', *Irish Medical Journal*, vol. 113 (2020), p. 24 (http://imj.ie/albrecht-von-graefes-ophthalmic-educa-tional-visit-to-william-wilde-in-dublin-in-1851/).

6   T.G. Wilson, *Victorian Doctor: Being the Life of Sir William Wilde* (2nd edn) (London: Methuen, 1942), pp 208, 212; M.T. Watts, 'Sir William Wilde 1815–1876: royal ophthalmologist extraordinary', *Journal of the Royal Society of Medicine*, vol. 83 (1990), pp 183–4 (https://doi.org/10.1177/014107689008300318).

7   W. Donnelly and W.R. Wilde, *The Census of Ireland for the Year 1851, Part V: Tables of Deaths. Volume I, Containing the Report, Tables of Pestilences, and Analysis of the Tables of Deaths* (Dublin: Alexander Thom and Sons, for Her Majesty's Stationery Office, 1856).

8   P. Froggatt, 'The demographic work of Sir William Wilde', *Irish Journal of Medical Science*, vol. 5 (1965), pp 213–30 (https://doi.org/10.1007/BF02943104).

9   S. Mullaney, 'Sir William Wilde and provision for the blind in nineteenth-century Ireland', *Irish Journal of Medical Science*, vol. 185 (2016), pp 281–3 (https://doi.org/10.1007/s11845-016-1434-6).

10 W.R. Wilde, *On the Physical, Moral, and Social Condition of the Deaf and Dumb* (London: John Churchill, 1854), pp 27, 30.

11 *Ibid.*, pp 6–7.

12 M. Walsh, 'William Wilde: his contribution to otology', *Irish Journal of Medical Science*, vol. 185 (2016), pp 291–2 (https://doi.org/10.1007/s11845-016-1435-5).

13 Wilde, *On the Physical, Moral, and Social Condition of the Deaf and Dumb*, p. 5.

14 *Ibid.*, pp 62–4.

15 J.B. Lyons, 'Sir William Wilde's medico-legal observations', *Medical History*, vol. 42 (1997), pp 437–54 (https://doi.org/10.1017/s0025727300063031).

16 M. O'Doherty, 'Sir William Wilde: an enlightened editor', *Irish Journal of Medical Science*, vol. 185 (2016), pp 297–9 (https://doi.org/10.1007/s11845-016-1437-3).

17 W.R. Wilde, 'The editor's preface: The history of periodic medical literature in Ireland, including notices of the medical and philosophical societies of Dublin', *Dublin Quarterly Journal of Medical Science*, vol. 1 (1846), pp i–xlviii (https://doi.org/10.1007/BF02995525).

18 W.R. Wilde, 'Report upon the recent epidemic fever in Ireland', *Dublin Quarterly Journal of Medical Science*, vol. 7 (1849), pp 64–126 (https://doi.org/10.1007/BF02949643); 'Report upon the recent epidemic fever in Ireland', *Dublin Quarterly Journal of Medical Science*, vol. 7 (1849), pp 340–404 (https://doi.org/10.1007/BF02953227); 'Report upon the recent epidemic fever in Ireland', *Dublin Quarterly Journal of Medical Science*, vol. 8 (1849), pp 1–86 (https://doi.org/10.1007/BF03021167); 'Report upon the recent epidemic fever in Ireland', *Dublin Quarterly Journal of Medical Science*, vol. 8 (1849), pp 270–339 (https://doi.org/10.1007/BF02961754); L. Geary, 'William Wilde: historian', *Irish Journal of Medical Science*, vol. 185 (2016), pp 301–2 (https://doi.org/10.1007/s11845-016-1427-5).

19 D. Coakley, 'William Wilde in the west of Ireland', *Irish Journal of Medical Science*, vol. 185 (2016), pp 277–80 (https://doi.org/10.1007/s11845-016-1433-7).

20 W.R. Wilde, 'Memoir of Gabriel Beranger, and his labours in the cause of Irish art, literature, and antiquities, from 1760 to 1780,

with illustrations', *Journal of the Royal Historical and Archaeological Association of Ireland*, vol. 1 (1870), pp 33–64, 121–52, 236–60 (http://www.jstor.org/stable/25506575).

21   W.R. Wilde, *Memoir of Gabriel Beranger and His Labours in the Cause of Irish Art and Antiquities from 1760 to 1780* (Dublin: Gill and Son, 1880).

22   *Ibid.*, p. 1.

23   R. Ellmann, *Oscar Wilde* (New York: Vintage Books, 1988), pp 14–15.

24   E. O'Sullivan, *The Fall of the House of Wilde* (London: Bloomsbury, 2016), pp 117–18.

25   D. Coakley, *Oscar Wilde: The Importance of Being Irish* (Dublin: Town House, 1994), pp 87–8.

26   M. Sturgis, *Oscar: A Life* (London: Apollo/Head of Zeus, 2018), p. 22.

27   G. Hanberry, *More Lives Than One: The Remarkable Wilde Family through the Generations* (Cork: Collins Press, 2011), pp 143–6.

28   E. McLysaght, 'Please stop acting as if liking coffee is a personality trait', *Irish Times*, 11 September 2021.

29   Part of this passage appeared as B.D. Kelly, 'Coffee, travel, and Sir William Wilde', *Medical Independent*, 7 February 2023 (https://www.medicalindependent.ie/comment/opinion/coffee-travel-and-sir-william-wilde/). It is reproduced and adapted by kind permission of GreenCross Publishing.

30   B. Kempton, *Wabi Sabi: Japanese Wisdom for a Perfectly Imperfect Life* (London: Piatkus, 2018).

31   H. Kuchler, 'Scientists battle to see off long Covid crisis', *Financial Times*, 5 January 2022.

32   A. Tait, 'Hope, high prices and long Covid', *The Observer*, 2 January 2022.

33   H. McGee, 'Estimated 114,000 may suffer long Covid', *Irish Times*, 28 January 2022; E. O'Regan, 'Suggestion 114,500 people have long Covid is an "underestimate"', *Irish Independent*, 29 January 2022.

34   'Facing up to long COVID', *The Lancet*, vol. 396 (2020), p. 1861 (https://doi.org/10.1016/S0140-6736(20)32662-3); 'And now for the aftershock', *The Economist,* 1 May 2021.

35   National Institute for Health and Care Excellence (NICE), Scottish Intercollegiate Guidelines Network (SIGN) and Royal College of

General Practitioners (RCGP), *COVID-19 Rapid Guideline: Managing the Long-Term Effects of COVID-19* (London: NICE, 2021), p. 5.

36　E. Mahase, 'Covid-19: what do we know about "long covid"?', *BMJ*, vol. 370 (2020), m2815 (https://doi.org/10.1136/bmj.m2815).

37　Part of this passage is adapted from B.D. Kelly and G. Gulati, 'The psychiatric impact of post-Covid-19 syndrome', *Update: Psychiatry and Neurology*, vol. 8 (2022), pp 34–5; B.D. Kelly and G. Gulati, 'The psychiatric impact of post-Covid-19 syndrome', *Medical Independent*, 24 February 2022 (https://www.medicalindependent.ie/clinical-news/psychiatry/the-psychiatric-impact-of-post-covid-19-syndrome/). It is adapted and reused here by kind permission of GreenCross Publishing and Professor Gautam Gulati.

38　P. Cullen, 'Coronavirus linked to elevated risk of mental health disorders', *Irish Times*, 17 February 2022.

39　B.D. Kelly and G. Gulati, 'Long COVID: the elephant in the room', *QJM*, vol. 115 (2022), pp 5–6 (https://doi.org/10.1093/qjmed/hcab299).

40　O. Moreno-Pérez, E. Merino, J.-M. Leon-Ramirez *et al.*, 'Post-acute COVID-19 syndrome. Incidence and risk factors: a Mediterranean cohort study', *Journal of Infection*, vol. 82 (2021), pp 373–8 (https://doi.org/10.1016/j.jinf.2021.01.004).

41　See https://www.yourcovidrecovery.nhs.uk/managing-the-effects/effects-on-your-body/taste-and-smell/.

42　B. Khraisat, A. Toubasi, L. AlZoubi, T. Al-Sayegh and A. Mansour, 'Meta-analysis of prevalence: the psychological sequelae among COVID-19 survivors', *International Journal of Psychiatry in Clinical Practice*, vol. 26 (2022), pp 234–43 (https://doi.org/10.1080/13651501.2021.1993924).

43　B.D. Kelly, *The Science of Happiness: The Six Principles of a Happy Life and the Seven Strategies for Achieving it* (Dublin: Gill Books, 2021), pp 101–23.

44　M. Taquet, J.R. Geddes, M. Husain, S. Luciano and P.J. Harrison, '6-month neurological and psychiatric outcomes in 236 379 survivors of COVID-19: a retrospective cohort study using electronic health records', *Lancet Psychiatry*, vol. 8 (2021), pp 416–27 (https://doi.org/10.1016/S2215-0366(21)00084-5).

45 G. Winter, 'Long Covid is "urgent" issue with "lingering psychological effects"', *Irish Times*, 11 January 2022.

46 M. Taquet, S. Luciano, J.-R. Geddes and P.J. Harrison, 'Bidirectional associations between COVID-19 and psychiatric disorder: retrospective cohort studies of 62354 COVID-19 cases in the USA', *Lancet Psychiatry*, vol. 8 (2021), pp 130–40 (https://doi.org/10.1016/S2215-0366(20)30462-4).

47 See also D. Huremović (ed.), *Psychiatry of Pandemics: A Mental Health Response to Infection Outbreak* (Cham: Springer, 2019).

48 V. Higgins, D. Sohaei, E.P. Diamandis and I. Prassas, 'COVID-19: from an acute to chronic disease? Potential long-term health consequences', *Critical Reviews in Clinical Laboratory Sciences*, vol. 58 (2021), pp 297–310 (https://doi.org/10.1080/10408363.2020.1860895).

49 'Omicron causes a less severe illness than earlier variants', *The Economist*, 1 January 2022.

50 E. Graham-Harrison, 'China sticks to zero Covid policy—but how long can isolation last?', *The Observer*, 2 January 2022 (https://www.theguardian.com/world/2022/jan/01/china-zero-covid-strategy-beijing-policy-protecting-public-health-coronavirus [courtesy of *Guardian* News & Media Ltd]).

51 See https://merrionstreet.ie/en/news-room/speeches/address_to_the_nation_taoiseach_michel_martin_td_21st_january_2022.html.

52 P. Leahy, J. Horgan-Jones and C. McQuinn, 'Emergency over', *Irish Times*, 22 and 23 January 2022.

53 K. Doyle, 'A new beginning', *Irish Independent*, 22 January 2022.

54 M. Paul, 'Good riddance to the Covid restrictions', *Irish Times*, 4 February 2022.

55 M. McCarthy, 'As soon as we get the official nod to ditch the masks, I will be ripping mine off', *Irish Independent*, 19 February 2022.

56 Some of this passage previously appeared as a blogpost I wrote for *Psychology Today*: B.D. Kelly, 'Giving thanks in the time of Covid-19 (Blogpost)', *Psychology Today*, 25 April 2020 (https://www.psychologytoday.com/ie/blog/psychiatry-and-society/202004/giving-thanks-in-the-time-covid-19 [© Brendan Kelly]). It is reused and adapted here by permission.

57 N. O'Leary, 'Is this the end of the pandemic?', *Irish Times*, 12 February 2022.

58   P. Cullen, 'Curing our health system from Covid', *Irish Times*, 29
      January 2022.

59   J. Hunt, 'The future of work', *Irish Times*, 23 April 2022.

60   C. Coleman, *News from Under a Coat Stand. A Diary, March–June
      2020* (Cork: Orla Kelly Publishing, 2021), p. 94. See also B.-H.
      Lévy, *The Virus in the Age of Madness* (New Haven and London: Yale
      University Press, 2020), pp 63–4; J. Farrar and A. Ahuja, *Spike: The
      Virus vs the People. The Inside Story* (paperback edn) (London: Profile
      Books, 2022), pp 141, 172, 174.

61   M. McCarthy, 'Working from home has its benefits—but we badly
      miss that daily human connection', *Irish Independent*, 31 August 2021.

62   J. Meagher, 'Generation Precarious: no security in work, at home or
      for old age', *Irish Independent*, 17 July 2021.

63   See https://president.ie/en/diary/details/president-speaks-at-the-an-
      nual-congress-of-the-european-federation-of-public-service-unions/
      speeches (© 2019 President of Ireland).

64   Defalque and Wright, 'Travers vs. Wilde and other: chloroform
      acquitted'.

65   W.R. Wilde, *Lough Corrib, its Shores and Islands: with Notices of Lough
      Mask* (Dublin: McGlashan and Gill, 1867).

66   *Ibid.*, p. 51.

67   *Ibid.*, pp 279–80.

68   P. Boland and S.P. Hughes, 'The enigma of Sir William Robert Wills
      Wilde (1815–1876)', *Journal of Medical Biography*, 21 October 2021
      (https://doi.org/10.1177/09677720211046588 [Epub ahead of print]).

69   P. Colum, *Moytura: A Play for Dancers* (Dublin: Dolmen Press, 1963);
      Wilson, *Victorian Doctor*.

70   E. Lou, *Field Notes from a Pandemic: A Journey through a World
      Suspended* (Toronto: Signal/McClelland and Stewart/Penguin
      Random House Canada, 2020), p. 37.

5. SPRING 2022: RESOLUTION

1   See www.rcpi.ie/heritage-centre.

2   'Wilde, Sir William', Kirkpatrick Index, RCPI Archive. I am very
      grateful to the RCPI Archive for this letter.

3 C. Lee, 'Chairman's opening address at the Sir William Wilde bi-centenary symposium', *Irish Journal of Medical Science*, vol. 185 (2016), pp 275–6 (https://doi.org/10.1007/s11845-016-1432-8).

4 See https://www.rcpi.ie/news/releases/capturing-covid-19-we-need-your-help-creating-a-pandemic-archive/.

5 J. Ganesh, 'Resist a false divination from the Covid crisis', *Financial Times*, 30 December 2020.

6 M. Honigsbaum, 'The silent killer we should have seen coming', *The Observer*, 21 June 2020.

7 B.D. Kelly, 'Between hope and despair, we must try to hold the line in the face of the coronavirus', *Irish Independent*, 31 October 2020.

8 See, for example, M. Lewis, *The Premonition: A Pandemic Story* (London: Allen Lane, 2021); M. Woolhouse, *The Year the World Went Mad: A Scientific Memoir* (Muir of Ord: Sandstone Press, 2022).

9 C. Colvin and E. McLaughlin, 'Revisiting the demography of the 1918 influenza pandemic in Ireland', *History Ireland*, vol. 29 (5) (2021), pp 38–41.

10 F. Zakaria, *Ten Lessons for a Post-Pandemic World* (London: Allen Lane, 2020).

11 R. Henderson, *Reimagining Capitalism in a World on Fire* (London: Penguin Business, 2021), p. xi.

12 G. Brown, *Seven Ways to Change the World: How to Fix the Most Pressing Problems We Face* (London: Simon and Schuster, 2021).

13 M. Carney, *Value(s): Building a Better World for All* (London: William Collins, 2021), p. 522.

14 S. Galloway, *Post Corona: From Crisis to Opportunity* (London: Bantam Press, 2020), p. 211.

15 A. Rajan (ed.), *Rethink: Leading Voices on Life After Crisis and How We Can Make a Better World* (London: BBC Books, 2021).

16 B.D. Kelly, 'Mental health and Covid-19: what can we do?', *Irish Pharmacy News*, November 2020.

17 J. Connell, 'Our souls need to catch up after a journey of lockdown before we can savour freedom', *Irish Independent*, 28 January 2022.

18 L. Neylon, 'In Phibsborough, a park that's always been locked may soon open', *Dublin Inquirer*, April 2022.

19 W. Donnelly and W.R. Wilde, *The Census of Ireland for the Year 1851, Part V: Tables of Deaths. Volume I, Containing the Report, Tables of*

Pestilences, and Analysis of the Tables of Deaths (Dublin: Alexander Thom and Sons, for Her Majesty's Stationery Office, 1856), p. 67 (hereafter *Tables of Deaths*).

20 *Ibid.*

21 *Ibid.*, p. 78.

22 *Ibid.*, p. 173.

23 C. Murphy, 'Pandemic arguments echo through the ages', *Sunday Independent*, 1 May 2022; M. Brennan, 'Finding cure for past plagues gives us hope for the future', *Irish Examiner*, 29 April 2022.

24 *Tables of Deaths*, pp 173–4 (Dr O'Brien 'refers to Mr Ball's recently published tract').

25 B. Gates, *How to Prevent the Next Pandemic* (London: Allen Lane, 2022).

26 D. Waltner-Toews, *On Pandemics: Deadly Diseases from Bubonic Plague to Coronavirus* (Vancouver and Berkeley: Greystone Books, 2020), pp 233–4.

27 'Battling the superbugs', *The Economist*, 22 January 2022.

28 D. Sridhar, *Preventable: How a Pandemic Changed the World and How to Stop the Next One* (London: Viking, 2022), p. 301.

29 B.D. Kelly, 'Pandemic is unfair, not NPHET or the Government', *Irish Times*, 13 July 2021.

30 J. Horgan-Jones and H. O'Connell, *Pandemonium: Power, Politics and Ireland's Pandemic* (Dublin: Gill Books, 2022), pp 330–1.

31 COVID-19 Excess Mortality Collaborators, 'Estimating excess mortality due to the COVID-19 pandemic: a systematic analysis of COVID-19-related mortality, 2020–21', *The Lancet*, vol. 399 (2022), pp 1513–36 (https://doi.org/10.1016/S0140-6736(21)02796-3).

32 E. O'Regan, 'Covid-19 impact below EU average', *Irish Examiner*, 8 April 2022; S. Collins, 'Appointment of Holohan a political molehill', *Irish Times*, 15 April 2022.

33 'Ireland's Covid restrictions now second lightest in the world', *Irish Times*, 27 March 2022.

34 P. Belluck, 'Do vaccines protect against long-term Covid symptoms?', *New York Times International Edition*, 28 April 2022; J. O'Connell, 'Covid has taught our health system nothing', *Irish Times*, 26 March 2022; P. Cullen, 'Latest Covid wave catches us off guard', *Irish Times*, 26 March 2022.

35   K. Hayhoe, *Saving Us: A Climate Scientist's Case for Hope and Healing in a Divided World* (New York: One Signal Publishers/Atria, 2021).

36   J. Watts, 'Climate crisis: The virus gave us a chance to change. Are we taking it?', *The Guardian*, 30 December 2020 (https://www.theguardian.com/world/2020/dec/29/could-covid-lockdown-have-helped-save-the-planet [courtesy of *Guardian* News & Media Ltd]). See also 'The new normal', *The Economist*, 18 December 2021.

37   B.D. Kelly, 'Tenacity of the human spirit', *Irish Times*, 12 May 2020.

38   E. Freud (ed.), *Letters of Sigmund Freud, Selected and Edited by Ernst Freud, 1873–1939* (New York: Dover Publications, 1960), pp 327–8. See also https://www.freud-museum.at/en/blog-posts-details/articles/freud-spanish-flu-and-covid-19.

39   S. Freud, 'Civilization and its Discontents (1929/30)', in *The Standard Edition of the Complete Psychological Works of Sigmund Freud, Volume XXI (1927–1931)* (London: Vintage, Hogarth Press and Institute of Psycho-Analysis, 2001), p. 93.

40   S. Freud, 'Delusions and Dreams in Jensen's *Gradiva* (1906/7)', in *The Standard Edition of the Complete Psychological Works of Sigmund Freud, Volume IX (1906–1908)* (London: Vintage, Hogarth Press and Institute of Psycho-Analysis, 2001), p. 22.

41   J. McGeachie, 'Wilde's worlds: Sir William Wilde in Victorian Ireland', *Irish Journal of Medical Science*, vol. 185 (2016), pp 303–7 (https://doi.org/10.1007/s11845-016-1428-4).

42   *Tables of Deaths*, pp 194–5.

43   D. Spiegelhalter and A. Masters, *Covid by Numbers: Making Sense of the Pandemic with Data* (London: Pelican Books, 2021).

44   D. Spiegelhalter and A. Masters, 'Can you capture the complex reality of the pandemic with numbers? Well, we tried …', *The Observer*, 2 January 2022 (https://www.theguardian.com/commentisfree/2022/jan/02/2021-year-when-interpreting-covid-statistics-crucial-to-reach-truth [courtesy of *Guardian* News & Media Ltd]).

45   M. Marshall, 'How can we end the pandemic?', *New Scientist*, vol. 253 (2022), pp 12–15.

46   R. Glynn, 'Think of vaccination as an added safety feature against Covid', *Irish Examiner*, 13 August 2021.

47   C. Cookson, A. Gross, N. Asgari and J. Cameron-Chileshe, 'How to reach the unvaccinated', *Financial Times*, 12 August 2021.

48   A. Ahuja, 'Lessons on how to live with Covid-19 are still to be learnt', *Financial Times*, 8/9 January 2022.

49   See, for example, L. O'Neill, *Keep Calm and Trust the Science: An Extraordinary Year in the Life of an Immunologist* (Dublin: Gill Books, 2021).

50   M. Scriven, E. Geary and B.D. Kelly, 'Psychiatrists and COVID-19: what is our role during this unprecedented time?', *Irish Journal of Psychological Medicine*, vol. 38 (2021), pp 307–12 (https://doi.org/10.1017/ipm.2020.95).

51   R. Bentall, 'Has the pandemic really caused a "tsunami" of mental health problems?', *The Guardian*, 9 February 2021.

52   L. Freeman, 'A year of Covid lessons from a monk's cloistered cell', *Financial Times*, 3/4 April 2021.

53   C. Murphy, 'Can we stop "living" Covid morning, noon and night—and just live with it?', *Sunday Independent*, 28 November 2021; E. O'Malley, 'Broadcast media obsession with daily Covid stats is self-serving', *Sunday Independent*, 28 November 2021.

54   E. Walshe, *The Diary of Mary Travers: A Novel* (Bantry: Somerville Press, 2014).

55   See www.rte.ie/news/leinster/2021/0325/1206152-violet-gibson-plaque and www.irishcentral.com/news/irish-woman-shot-mussolini-plaque-dublin.

56   A version of this passage was first published as B.D. Kelly, 'The woman who shot Mussolini', *Medical Independent*, 27 January 2022. It is adapted and reused here by kind permission of GreenCross Publishing.

57   F. Stonor Saunders, *The Woman Who Shot Mussolini* (London: Faber and Faber, 2010).

58   See https://councilmeetings.dublincity.ie/mgAi.aspx?ID=22326.

59   A. Camus, *La Peste (The Plague)* (Paris: Gallimard, 1947).

60   R.A. Higgins, *Pathogens Love a Patsy: Pandemic and Other Poems* (Cliffs of Moher: Salmon Poetry, 2020); C. Fitzpatrick, *Poetic Licence in a Time of Corona* (Dublin: Twenty First Century Renaissance, 2022).

61   S. Sontag, *Illness as Metaphor* (New York: Farrar, Straus and Giroux, 1978).

62 H.B. Levine and A. de Staal (eds), *Psychoanalysis and Covidian Life: Common Distress, Individual Experience* (Bicester: Phoenix Publishing House, 2021).

63 See https://president.ie/en/diary/details/president-gives-an-address-at-the-scientific-council-of-the-european-resear/speeches (© 2016 President of Ireland).

64 See https://president.ie/en/media-library/speeches/the-future-of-europe-re-balancing-ecology-economics-and-ethics-lecture-by-michael-d-higgins-president-of-ireland (© 2019 President of Ireland).

65 Part of this passage previously appeared as a blogpost I wrote for *Psychology Today*: B.D. Kelly, 'What we've lost, how we'll recover (Blogpost)', *Psychology Today*, 20 May 2020 (https://www.psychologytoday.com/ie/blog/psychiatry-and-society/202005/what-weve-lost-how-well-recover [© Brendan Kelly]). It is reused and adapted here by permission.

66 B.D. Kelly, 'The five stages of Covid's psychological impact', *Irish Independent*, 27 February 2021.

67 B.D. Kelly, 'Quarantine, restrictions and mental health in the COVID-19 pandemic', *QJM*, vol. 114 (2021), pp 93–4 (https://doi.org/10.1093/qjmed/hcaa322).

68 B.D. Kelly, 'Despite all that's going wrong in the world, we are still a pretty happy bunch', *Irish Independent*, 1 April 2021; H. Mance, 'Happiness can still be found during the crisis', *Financial Times*, 30/31 January 2021.

69 E. Kübler-Ross, *On Death and Dying* (New York: Macmillan, 1969).

70 B.D. Kelly, *The Doctor Who Sat for a Year* (Dublin: Gill Books, 2019), pp 76–7.

71 N.A. Christakis, *Apollo's Arrow: The Profound and Enduring Impact of Coronavirus on the Way We Live* (New York: Little, Brown Spark, 2020), p. 324. See also 'The big picture', *The Economist*, 2 January 2021.

72 'The triumph of big government', *The Economist*, 20 November 2021.

73 S. Reicher, 'No. 10's opacity is corrosive. We need openness', *The Guardian*, 13 May 2020 (https://www.theguardian.com/commentisfree/2020/may/13/british-people-lockdown-coronavirus-crisis [courtesy of *Guardian* News & Media Ltd]).

74 Y.N. Harari, 'The Covid year', *Financial Times*, 27/28 February 2021.

75 A. Staines and D. Carey, '"Living with Covid" is empty sloganeering in need of a plan', *Irish Times*, 16 May 2022.

76 D. McWilliams, 'We are entering the Roaring Twenties', *Irish Times*, 31 July 2021.

77 D. MacKenzie, *Stopping the Next Pandemic: How Covid-19 Can Help Us Save Humanity* (London: Bridge Street Press, 2020), pp 300–1.

78 See https://www.president.ie/en/media-library/speeches/speech-at-at-the-launch-of-the-first-thought-talks-strand-of-galway-interna (© 2018 President of Ireland).

79 See https://www.president.ie/en/media-library/speeches/ireland-and-lithuania-towards-a-shared-future-within-the-european-union (© 2018 President of Ireland).

80 R. Harding, 'Human progress stumbles on, Covid or no Covid', *Financial Times*, 22 December 2021.

81 B.D. Kelly, 'Politicians are as important as doctors for Covid recovery', *Sunday Times*, 22 November 2020.

82 L. Geddes, 'Having Covid-19 linked to risk of economic hardship, study suggests', *The Guardian*, 9 March 2022 (https://www.theguardian.com/society/2022/mar/09/covid-19-risk-economic-hardship-poverty-study-suggests [courtesy of *Guardian* News & Media Ltd]).

83 L. Spinney, '"We must revive the social state". Pandemics can lead to equality, suggests Piketty', *The Guardian*, 13 May 2020 (https://www.theguardian.com/world/2020/may/12/will-coronavirus-lead-to-fairer-societies-thomas-piketty-explores-the-prospect).

84 B.D. Kelly, *Coping with Coronavirus. How to Stay Calm and Protect Your Mental Health: A Psychological Toolkit* (Newbridge: Merrion Press, 2020).

85 S. Carey, 'Personal power to create positive outlook can change paradigm and reduce isolation', *Irish Independent*, 26 February 2022.

86 C. Cavendish, 'Britain's youngsters are scarred by post-pandemic anxiety', *Financial Times*, 26/27 February 2022.

87 S. Taylor, 'I wrote the book on pandemic psychology. Post-Covid will take some getting used to', *The Guardian*, 24 February 2022 (https://www.theguardian.com/commentisfree/2022/feb/24/pandemic-psychology-end-covid-pandemic-normal).

88   A. Gross, 'History shows pandemics rarely end neatly or with complete eradication', *Financial Times*, 13/14 March 2021.

89   M. Ignatieff, *On Consolation: Finding Solace in Dark Times* (New York: Metropolitan Books, 2021).

90   See https://president.ie/en/diary/details/president-hosts-a-reception-commemorating-the-great-flu-epidemic-of-1918-1919/speeches (© 2019 President of Ireland).

EPILOGUE

1   M. McCarthy, 'Learning to roll with the disappointments will make travel and holidays much easier', *Irish Independent*, 2 June 2022.

2   B. Cunningham, *Medieval Irish Pilgrims to Santiago de Compostela* (Dublin: Four Courts Press, 2018).

3   P. Coelho, *The Pilgrimage: A Contemporary Quest for Ancient Wisdom* (New York: Harper, 2004).

4   S. MacLaine, *The Camino: A Pilgrimage of Courage* (London: Pocket Books, 2001).

5   B. Chermisde, *The Only Way is West: A Once in a Lifetime Adventure Walking 500 Miles on Spain's Camino de Santiago* (Wrocław: Amazon, 2019).

6   Filmax and Elixir Films, 2010.

7   P. French, '*The Way*—review', *The Observer*, 15 May 2011 (https://www.theguardian.com/film/2011/may/15/the-way-emilio-estevez-martin-sheen-review).

8   R. Williams, 'Modern-day pilgrims beat a path to the Camino', *The Guardian*, 2 May 2011 (https://www.theguardian.com/travel/2011/may/02/camino-pilgrims-route [courtesy of *Guardian* News & Media Ltd]).

9   H. Kerkeling, *I'm Off Then: Losing and Finding Myself on the Camino de Santiago* (New York: Free Press, 2009).

10   *Ich Bin Dann Mal Weg*, directed by Julia von Heinz and starring Devid Striesow as Hape Kerkeling (Gesellschaft für feine Filme and UFA Fiction, 2015).

11 S. Ramis, *Camino de Santiago (Revised and Updated)* (London: Aurum Press, 2017); J. Brierley, *Camino de Santiago: St. Jean Pied de Port–Santiago de Compostela: Maps* (Dyke: Camino Guides, 2019).

12 See www.rte.ie/news/coronavirus/2022/0511/1297345-coronavirus-travel.

13 W.R. Wilde, *Narrative of a Voyage to Madeira, Teneriffe, and Along the Shores of the Mediterranean, Including a Visit to Algiers, Egypt, Palestine, Tyre, Rhodes, Telmessus, Cyprus, and Greece, with Observations on the Present State and Prospects of Egypt and Palestine, and on the Climate, Natural History, Antiquities, etc. of the Countries Visited* (Dublin: William Curry, 1840), p. 230.

14 P. Stanford, 'Secular pilgrims: why ancient trails still pack a spiritual punch', *The Observer*, 28 March 2021 (https://www.theguardian.com/lifeandstyle/2021/mar/28/secular-pilgrims-why-ancient-trails-still-pack-a-spiritual-punch [courtesy of *Guardian* News & Media Ltd]).

INDEX

NB Mc is treated as Mac; St is treated as Saint.